STUDY GUIDE
TO ESSENTIALS OF
CLINICAL PSYCHIATRY

BASED ON

THE AMERICAN PSYCHIATRIC PRESS
TEXTBOOK OF PSYCHIATRY, THIRD EDITION

STUDY GUIDE TO ESSENTIALS OF CLINICAL PSYCHIATRY

BASED ON

THE AMERICAN PSYCHIATRIC PRESS
TEXTBOOK OF PSYCHIATRY, THIRD EDITION

DONALD M. HILTY, M.D.
Assistant Professor of Clinical Psychiatry,
University of California, Davis School of Medicine,
Sacramento, California

ROBERT E. HALES, M.D., M.B.A.
Professor and Chair, Department of Psychiatry,
University of California, Davis School of Medicine;
Director, Behavioral Health Center, UC Davis Health System;
Medical Director, Sacramento County Mental Health Services,
Sacramento, California

STUART C. YUDOFSKY, M.D.
D. C. and Irene Ellwood Professor and Chairman,
Department of Psychiatry and Behavioral Sciences,
Baylor College of Medicine; Chief, Psychiatry Service,
The Methodist Hospital, Houston, Texas

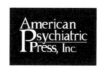

American Psychiatric Press, Inc.

Washington, DC
London, England

Copyright 1999 American Psychiatric Press, Inc.

02 01 00 99 4 3 2 1

First Edition

ALL RIGHTS RESERVED

Manufactured in the United States of America on acid-free paper

American Psychiatric Press, Inc.

1400 K Street, N.W.

Washington, DC 20005

www.appi.org

CONTENTS

PREFACE

T he *Study Guide to Essentials of Clinical Psychiatry* is written principally to accompany *Essentials of Clinical Psychiatry*, but, as the reader will learn, may also be used by purchasers of the *Textbook of Psychiatry*, Third Edition. The *Textbook of Psychiatry*, Third Edition is a clinically focused, one-volume, comprehensive, and up-to-date textbook designed for psychiatrists, psychiatry residents, and other mental health professionals desiring a reference book for the field of psychiatry. *Essentials of Clinical Psychiatry* is a synopsis of the Textbook designed specifically for senior medical students; residents in psychiatry, neurology, and primary care; and practicing physicians in these fields and other specialties desiring a clinically focused psychiatry text. *Essentials of Clinical Psychiatry* contains the 25 most clinically relevant chapters from the third edition of the Textbook and presents these chapters in a condensed manner that facilitates learning and applications of concepts to patient care. The purpose of the Study Guide is to provide readers of the Textbook and the Essentials with an opportunity to evaluate their understanding of materials taken from sections on theoretical foundations, assessment issues, psychiatric disorders, psychiatric treatments, and special topics.

For the first time, the Study Guide can be used by readers for both the Textbook and the Essentials. Previous editions of the Study Guide were based on the extensive material in the Textbook, which render many questions unhelpful for readers of the Essentials. In fact, the current edition of the Study Guide was distilled to 25 chapters of questions to correspond exactly to the chapters in the Essentials. This was done because the readers most likely to use the Study Guide and Essentials are medical students and residents in psychiatry, neurology, and primary care, and psychiatrists and neurologists preparing for their specialty board examinations. The Study Guide is still applicable to the most important chapters of the Textbook, because the Essentials is distilled from the Textbook, and complete answers are included for each question so the reader does not have to return to either book to learn why the answer was selected.

The Study Guide has also been improved by adjusting the number of questions per chapter to coincide with the amount of material contained in the chapters in the Essentials. In past editions of the Study Guide, each chapter contained 10 questions that failed to discriminate between topics that have been well researched and described (e.g., mood disorders) from topics with less empirical information available (e.g., adjustment disorders). The current edition of the Study Guide has at least 10 questions in each chapter as before, but has up to 30 questions on key topics: "Mood Disorders," "Psychopharmacology," and "Disorders First Diagnosed in Infancy, Childhood, or Adolescence." The increased number of questions for these chapters will help readers to better evaluate their understanding of the material.

The Study Guide consists of approximately 95% new questions that were written to test readers on the most recent developments in the field as well as on key points contained within the literature. The new questions will also provide a renewed challenge to the readers of the second edition of the Textbook, the *Synopsis of Psychiatry*, and the previous Study Guide. Theoretically, avid medical students, residents, or clinicians could use both the current and previous editions of the Study Guide to prepare for examinations.

In summary, we hope that you will find the *Study Guide to Essentials of Clinical Psychiatry* to be a useful addition to your continuing education needs. We welcome comments and critiques of the Study Guide so that we may improve and streamline the next edition.

—*Donald M. Hilty, M.D.*
Robert E. Hales, M.D., M.B.A.
Stuart C. Yudofsky, M.D.

CHAPTER 1

THE NEUROSCIENTIFIC FOUNDATIONS OF PSYCHIATRY

QUESTIONS

Directions: Select the single best response for each of the following questions:

1.1   "Classical" neurotransmitters include all of the following **EXCEPT**
    A.   Norepinephrine.
    B.   Glycine.
    C.   Glutamic acid.
    D.   Acetylcholine.
    E.   *N*-acetylapartyglutamate.

1.2   The rate-limiting enzyme in catecholamine synthesis is
    A.   Tyrosine hydroxylase.
    B.   Dopa decarboxylase.
    C.   Dopamine β-hydroxylase.
    D.   Phenylethanolamine-*N*-methyltransferase.
    E.   None of the above.

1.3   The enzyme localized on the outer membrane of the mitochondria and that metabolizes catecholamines is
    A.   Protein kinase.
    B.   Monoamine oxidase (MAO).
    C.   Catechol-*O*-methyltransferase (COMT).
    D.   Acetylcholinesterase.
    E.   All of the above.

1.4   In many, if not most cases, a neuron may release
    A.   One neurotransmitter.
    B.   Two different neurotransmitters.

1

   C. Three different neurotransmitters.
   D. Four different neurotransmitters.
   E. Five different neurotransmitters.

1.5   Which of the following plays an important role in the ability of the nervous system to adapt to the environment?
   A. DNA polymorphisms.
   B. Protein phosphorylation.
   C. Protein transcription.
   D. All of the above.
   E. None of the above.

1.6   Which of the following is true?
   A. The 5-HT$_{1A}$ receptor is the site of action of the anxiolytic drug buspirone.
   B. The primary source of serotonergic innervation in the brain is the locus coeruleus.
   C. Agonists at the 5-HT$_3$ receptor reduce nausea.
   D. Antagonists at the 5-HT$_{1D}$ receptor reduce migraines.
   E. All of the above.

1.7   Which of the following is true?
   A. Neuropeptides are synthesized within the nerve terminal.
   B. Second messengers usually exert their main biological effects via protein kinases.
   C. Cholinergic drugs antagonize REM sleep, whereas anticholingeric drugs promote REM sleep.
   D. All of the above.
   E. None of the above.

1.8   The psychotomimetic effects of phencyclidine (PCP) are mediated by
   A. Glycine.
   B. Serotonin.
   C. Glutamate.
   D. Dopamine.
   E. Acetylcholine.

Directions: For each of the statements below, one or more of the answers is correct. Choose

   A. If 1, 2, and 3 are correct.
   B. If only 1 and 3 are correct.
   C. If only 2 and 4 are correct.

D. If only 4 is correct.

E. If all are correct.

1.9　When the neuronal membrane is depolarized,

1. Voltage-gated Na^+ channels open.
2. Na^+ flows out of the cell.
3. Voltage-gated Ca^{++} channels open in the presynaptic terminal in response to the arrival of the action potential.
4. Ca^{++} flows out of the cell.

1.10　Benzodiazepines are superior to barbiturates because they have

1. A more favorable ratio between anxiolytic action and sedative effects.
2. A greater therapeutic index.
3. Less risk for dependence.
4. Fewer serious withdrawal symptoms.

1.11　Which of the following is true?

1. Neurotransmitters are synthesized in the nerve terminal.
2. Neuropeptides are synthesized in the cell body.
3. Peptidergic neurons may be less rapidly responsive because supplemental neuropeptides must be transported from the perikaryon to the axon.
4. A single gene may give rise to multiple active peptides.

1.12　The major inhibitory transmitter

1. In the brain is γ-aminobutyric acid (GABA).
2. In the spinal cord is GABA.
3. Hyperpolarizes the neuronal membrane in the brain and spinal cord by influx of chloride.
4. Hyperpolarizes the neuronal membrane in the brain and spinal cord by influx of sodium.

1.13　Which of the following agents exert their effect via GABAergic neurons?

1. Benzodiazepines.
2. Anticonvulsants.
3. Barbiturates.
4. β-blockers.

1.14　The mechanism(s) by which antipsychotic medications are known to work include

1. Dopamine receptor blockade.
2. Altering proteins by second messengers.

     3.   Altering limbic neurotransmission.

     4.   Changes in gene expression.

1.15   Which of the following is true regarding the blockade of dopamine receptors?

     1.   Blockade in the arcuate nucleus increases prolactin levels.

     2.   Blockade in the ventral tegmental area may improve attention and cognition.

     3.   Blockade in the nigrostriatal pathway results in extrapyramidal side effects.

     4.   Blockade in the ventral tegmental area may increase craving associated with substance abuse.

ANSWERS

1.1   The answer is **E.** "Classical" neurotransmitters include all of the following except N-acetylapartyglutamate.

1.2   The answer is **A.** The rate-limiting enzyme in catecholamine synthesis is tyrosine hydroxylase.

1.3   The answer is **B.** The enzyme localized on the outer membrane of the mitochondria that metabolizes catecholamines is MAO. COMT, which also metabolizes catecholamines, is located in the extracellular space.

1.4   The answer is **B.** In many, if not most cases, a neuron may release two different neurotransmitters.

1.5   The answer is **B.** Protein phosphorylation, along with the regulation of gene expression, is the most significant mechanism involved in the regulation of long-term adaptation to the environment.

1.6   The answer is **A.** The 5-HT_{1A} receptor is the site of action of the anxiolytic drug buspirone. The primary source of serotonergic innervation in the brain is the raphe nucleus. *Antagonists* at the 5-HT_3 receptor reduce nausea. *Agonists* at the 5-HT_{1D} receptor reduce migraines.

1.7   The answer is **B.** Second messengers usually exert their main biological effects via protein kinases; however, there are some exceptions (e.g., cyclic AMP can independently gate certain ion channels in the olfactory system).

1.8   The answer is **C.** The psychotomimetic effects of PCP are mediated by glutamate.

1.9 The answer is **B.** When the neuronal membrane is depolarized voltage-gated Na^+ channels open and voltage-gated Ca^{++} channels open in the presynaptic terminal in response to the arrival of the action potential. Na^+ flows *into* the cell and Ca^{++} flows *into* the cell.

1.10 The answer is **E.** The benzodiazepines are superior to barbiturates because they have a more favorable ratio between anxiolytic action and sedative effects, a greater therapeutic index, less risk for dependence and fewer serious withdrawal symptoms.

1.11 The answer is **E.** Neurotransmitters are synthesized in the nerve terminal and neuropeptides are synthesized in the cell body. Peptidergic neurons may be less rapidly responsive because supplemental neuropeptides must be transported from the perikaryon to the axon. A single gene may give rise to multiple active peptides.

1.12 The answer is **B.** The major inhibitory transmitter in the brain is GABA. In the spinal cord, the major inhibitory transmitter is glycine. Both hyperpolarize the neuronal membrane by influx of chloride.

1.13 The answer is **A.** Benzodiazepines, anticonvulsants, and barbiturates exert their effect via GABAergic neurons. β-blockers exert their effect via noradrenergic neurons.

1.14 The answer is **E.** The mechanism(s) by which antipsychotic medications work include dopamine receptor blockade, altering proteins, altering limbic neurotransmission, and changes in gene expression.

1.15 The answer is **A.** Blockade in the arcuate nucleus increases prolactin levels. Blockade in the ventral tegmental area may improve attention and cognition. Blockade in the nigrostriatal pathway results in extrapyramidal side effects. Blockade in the ventral tegmental area may *reduce* craving associated with substance abuse.

CHAPTER 2

NORMAL CHILD AND ADOLESCENT DEVELOPMENT

QUESTIONS

Directions: Select the single best response for each of the following questions:

2.1 A child speaks with a 20- to 50-word vocabulary at approximately
   A. 6 months.
   B. 12 months.
   C. 18 months.
   D. 24 months.
   E. 30 months.

2.2 Epigenesis is a concept that
   A. States developmental steps occur sequentially.
   B. Freud developed to explain how conflict affects behavior.
   C. States resolution of prior experiences is required before one progresses to the next stage.
   D. States that development involves changing structures over time that permit alterations in organization that are not dependent on the outcome of prior stages.
   E. A and C.

2.3 Freud believed certain core issues were the source of anxiety and conflict in patients. In which order do these issues arise, according to Freud?
   A. Separation, helplessness, guilt, and castration.
   B. Helplessness, separation, castration, and guilt.
   C. Helplessness, castration, separation, and guilt.
   D. Guilt, helplessness, separation, and castration.
   E. Guilt, castration, separation, and helplessness.

2.4   Which of the following is **FALSE?**
   A.   At the sensory-motor stage, an infant is embedded in a trial-and-error world.
   B.   Reasoning begins during the sensory-motor stage.
   C.   Internalization of actions begins during the preoperational stage.
   D.   At the formal operational stage, the rules of logic of language are established.
   E.   None of the above.

2.5   An adult pattern of sleep is typically established on a physiological level by
   A.   6 months.
   B.   9 months.
   C.   12 months.
   D.   15 months.
   E.   18 months.

2.6   Which is true about puberty?
   A.   Menarche is frequently followed by irregular anovulatory periods for 12–18 months.
   B.   Females reach puberty before males.
   C.   Females have a height spurt before males.
   D.   Girls achieve menarche at a mean age of approximately 13 years.
   E.   All of the above.

2.7   A common psychological defense for adolescents is
   A.   Projection.
   B.   Isolation of affect.
   C.   Sublimation.
   D.   Regression.
   E.   None of the above.

2.8   The age at onset of stranger anxiety is typically
   A.   5 months.
   B.   7 months.
   C.   9 months.
   D.   11 months.
   E.   13 months.

2.9   Which of the following is true?
   A.   Wariness of strangers is apparent by 3 months.
   B.   Achievement of three- to six-word mean length of utterance is accomplished by 3 years of age.

    C. Females reach puberty 2 years earlier than males.

    D. All of the above.

    E. None of the above.

2.10   Castration anxiety occurs mainly between
    A. 2–4 years.
    B. 4–6 years.
    C. 6–8 years.
    D. 8–10 years.
    E. None of the above.

Directions: For each of the statements below, one or more of the answers is correct. Choose

    A. If 1, 2, and 3 are correct.
    B. If only 1 and 3 are correct.
    C. If only 2 and 4 are correct.
    D. If only 4 is correct.
    E. If all are correct.

2.11   Gesell's landmarks of normal behavioral development at 18 months include ability to
    1. Walk down stairs with one hand held.
    2. Spontaneously scribble.
    3. Use 20–29 words.
    4. Occasionally indicate toilet needs.

2.12   Which of the following is true regarding the sleep of children?
    1. Light sleep (Stages 1 and 2) dominates during the first 3 months of life.
    2. Premature infants spend 25% of their time in Stage 1 REM pattern.
    3. By 3 months of age, approximately 70% of babies become night sleepers, rescinding their pattern of waking at 3- to 4-hour intervals.
    4. By 6 months, the adult pattern of sleep is established.

2.13   By age 7, children begin to
    1. Understand that their feelings, intuitions, and thoughts may be of interest to others.
    2. Understand cause-and-effect relationships.
    3. Become rule bound and even moralistic about rules.
    4. Develop abstract intelligence.

2.14   Which of the following are considered developmental themes of adolescence?
1. Normalization versus privacy.
2. Idealization versus devaluation.
3. Dependence versus independence.
4. Trust versus mistrust.

2.15   Newborns
1. Scan faces like inanimate patterns.
2. Can discriminate between mother's voice from that of another woman reading the same material.
3. Seek out little sensory stimulation.
4. Are able to reliably imitate an adult model who smiled, frowned, or showed surprise.

ANSWERS

2.1   The answer is **C**. A child speaks with 20- to 50-word vocabulary at approximately 18 months.

2.2   The answer is **E**. Epigenesis is a concept that states sequential steps influence subsequent steps and resolution of prior experiences is required before one progresses to the next stage. Hierarchic reorganization is the concept that development involves changing structures over time that permit alterations in organization that are not dependent on the outcome of prior stages. Freud did not develop the idea of epigenesis.

2.3   The answer is **B**. Freud believed certain core issues were the source of anxiety and conflict in patients. The order in which these issues arise, according to Freud, is helplessness, separation, castration, and guilt.

2.4   The answer is **E**. All of the statements are true.

2.5   The answer is **C**. An adult pattern of sleep is typically established on a physiological level by 12 months.

2.6   The answer is **E**. All of the following are true about puberty: menarche is frequently followed by irregular anovulatory periods for 12–18 months; females reach puberty before males; females have a height spurt before males; and girls achieve menarche at a mean age of 12.7 years.

2.7 The answer is **A.** A common psychological defense for adolescents is projection.

2.8 The answer is **B.** The onset of stranger anxiety is typically 7 months.

2.9 The answer is **D.** All of the statements are correct.

2.10 The answer is **B.** Castration anxiety occurs mainly between 4–6 years.

2.11 The answer is **A.** Gesell's landmarks of normal behavioral development at 18 months include ability to walk down stairs with one hand held, spontaneously scribble, and use 20–29 words. Children usually indicate toilet needs around 24 months.

2.12 The answer is **B.** The following is true regarding the sleep of children: light sleep (Stages 1 and 2) dominates during the first 3 months of life and by 3 months of age, approximately 70% of babies become night sleepers, rescinding their pattern of waking at 3- to 4-hour intervals. Premature infants spend 75% of their time in Stage 1 REM pattern. By 12 months, the adult pattern of sleep is established.

2.13 The answer is **A.** By age seven, children begin to understand that their feelings, intuitions, and thoughts may be of interest to others, understand cause-and-effect relationships, and become rule bound and even moralistic about rules. They do not develop abstract intelligence until age 14.

2.14 The answer is **A.** Developmental themes of adolescence include normalization versus privacy, idealization versus devaluation, and dependence versus independence. Trust versus mistrust is a developmental theme characteristic of infancy according to Erikson.

2.15 The answer is **C.** Newborns can discriminate between mother's voice from that of another woman reading the same material and are able to reliably imitate an adult model who smiled, frowned, or showed surprise. They scan faces in a different way than inanimate patterns. They commonly seek out sensory stimulation.

CHAPTER 3
THEORIES OF THE MIND AND PSYCHOPATHOLOGY

QUESTIONS

Directions: Select the single best response for each of the following questions:

3.1   The topographical model of the mind is supported by
   A.   The fact that comatose patients can report registering events that took place while they had been unconscious.
   B.   The act of dreaming.
   C.   A slip of the tongue.
   D.   Resistance to remembering.
   E.   All of the above.

3.2   The defense mechanism of regression
   A.   Helps separate affect from memory.
   B.   Explains hand-washing secondary to fantasies of soiling.
   C.   Is not uncommon in medically ill patients.
   D.   Is invalidation of an unpleasant or unwanted piece of information.
   E.   None of the above.

3.3   Which of the following would be a clear example of projection?
   A.   "I hate him because he hates me."
   B.   "If I hate him, he will think I am a bad person."
   C.   "If he hates me, I should also hate him."
   D.   "I don't hate him, he hates me."
   E.   All of the above.

3.4   Melanie Klein's work focused on
   A.   The process of pathological identification and the fate of the incorporated selfobject.

B. The concept that the objects were primary and the drives were inter-changeable.

C. The concept of the cohesive self, which requires optimal empathy consist-ing of mirroring and idealization.

D. The concept of the "good enough" mother.

E. None of the above.

3.5   A developmental theory based on the phases of separation and individuation was proposed by

A. Abraham.

B. Adler.

C. Klein.

D. Kernberg.

E. Mahler.

3.6   In Erickson's model of development, a latency age child deals with

A. Trust versus mistrust.

B. Autonomy versus shame.

C. Initiative versus guilt.

D. Industry versus inferiority.

E. Intimacy versus isolation.

3.7   Dissociation is a defense mechanism that combines

A. Repression, regression, and isolation.

B. Denial, repression, and isolation.

C. Reaction formation, reversal, and repression.

D. Regression, turning against the self, and denial.

E. Isolation, splitting, and reaction formation.

3.8   Which of the following patients respond well to confrontation, according to Kernberg?

A. Narcissistic patients.

B. Borderline patients.

C. Both narcissistic and borderline patients.

D. Neither narcissistic or borderline patients.

3.9   When the characteristics of the parent become the child's own in a way that allows the child to modify them as he or she sees fit, it is called

A. Introjection.

B. Projection.

C. Identification.

D. Projective identification.
E. Repression.

Directions: For each of the statements below, one or more of the answers is correct. Choose

A. If 1, 2, and 3 are correct.
B. If only 1 and 3 are correct.
C. If only 2 and 4 are correct.
D. If only 4 is correct.
E. If all are correct.

3.10 Elements associated with primary process include
1. The pleasure principle.
2. Condensation.
3. Displacement.
4. Symbolization.

3.11 The death instinct consists of
1. Aggression and the tendency to create destruction and disorder.
2. The compulsion to repeat, even without constructive purpose.
3. The establishment of stimulus barriers to achieve a state of quiescence.
4. Aggressive instincts that function autonomously from sexual or erotic instincts.

3.12 Chronic trauma can lead to
1. Somatization.
2. Hypervigilance.
3. Incest.
4. Dissociation.

3.13 Object relations theory explains that
1. In secondary narcissism, the individual is concerned with and in love with him- or herself.
2. When we lose a close friend or family member to death, we mourn the loss in and of itself but also the loss of an object on which to project.
3. As children grow older, they no longer have any primary narcissism.
4. Unresolved trauma leads a person to depend on others for maintenance of self-esteem.

3.14   Which is true about the structural model of the mind?
   1.   The id forms an alliance with the ego.
   2.   The ego is not concerned with gratification.
   3.   The id wants gratification.
   4.   The ego can accomplish its goals without the help of the id.

3.15   Which of the following statements is true regarding the hypotheses of Freud and Jung?
   1.   Freud thought that libido was sexual, and Jung thought it was a unitary force of psychic energy (not explicitly sexual).
   2.   Freud believed the unconscious was the product of the individual's history, whereas Jung believed it was the product of both the personal history (minor part) and a collective history (major part).
   3.   Freud holds that the dream was the unique idiosyncratic product of the dreamer, whereas Jung contended it revealed imbalance in the unity of the self.
   4.   Freud posited that archetypes are autonomous, and Jung posited that archetypes are semiautonomous.

ANSWERS

3.1   The answer is **E.** The topographical model of the mind is supported by the fact that comatose patients can report registering events that took place while they had been unconscious, the act of dreaming, a slip of the tongue, and resistance to remembering.

3.2   The answer is **B.** Regression is not uncommon in medically ill patients. It does not help to separate affect from memory (isolation of affect), explain hand-washing secondary to fantasies of soiling (undoing), or invalidate an unpleasant or unwanted piece of information (denial).

3.3   The answer is **D.** A clear example of projection is the statement "I don't hate him, he hates me."

3.4   The answer is **A.** Melanie Klein's work focused on the process of pathological identification and to the fate of the incorporated selfobject. Others' work include the concept that the objects were primary and the drives were interchangeable (Fairbairn), the concept of the cohesive self, which requires optimal empathy consisting of mirroring and idealization (Kohut), and the concept of the "good enough" mother (Winnicott).

3.5　　The answer is **E.** A developmental theory based on the phases of separation and individuation was proposed by Mahler.

3.6　　The answer is **D.** In Erikson's model of development, a latency age child deals with industry versus inferiority.

3.7　　The answer is **B.** Dissociation is a defense mechanism that combines denial, repression, and isolation.

3.8　　The answer is **B.** Patients with borderline states respond well to confrontation according to Kernberg.

3.9　　The answer is **C.** When the characteristics of the parent become the child's own in a way that allows the child to modify them as he or she sees fit, it is called identification.

3.10　The answer is **E.** Elements associated with primary process include the pleasure principle, condensation, displacement, and symbolization.

3.11　The answer is **A.** The death instinct consists of aggression and the tendency to create destruction and disorder, the compulsion to repeat, even without constructive purpose, and the establishment of stimulus barriers to achieve a state of quiescence. Freud believed that aggressive instincts always function in concert with sexual or erotic instincts.

3.12　The answer is **C.** Chronic trauma can lead to hypervigilance and dissociation.

3.13　The answer is **C.** Object relations theory explains that when we lose a close friend or family member to death, we mourn the loss in and of itself but also the loss of an object on which to project. Unresolved trauma leads a person to depend on others for maintenance of self-esteem. In secondary narcissism, the individual makes choices of persons like him- or herself. As children grow older, they retain some reserve of primary narcissism to fuel self-esteem and self-confidence.

3.14　The answer is **B.** According to the structural model of the mind, the id forms an alliance with the ego and the id wants gratification. In addition, the ego *is* concerned with gratification, though less than the id, and cannot accomplish its goals without the help of the id.

3.15   The answer is **A.** Freud thought that libido was sexual, and Jung thought it was a unitary force of psychic energy (not explicitly sexual). Freud believed the unconscious was the product of the individual's history, whereas Jung believed it was the product of both the personal history (minor part) and a collective history (major part). Freud holds that the dream was the unique idiosyncratic product of the dreamer, whereas Jung contended it revealed imbalance in the unity of the self. Freud did *not* put forth any construct regarding archetypes, whereas Jung posited that they were semiautonomous.

CHAPTER 4

THE PSYCHIATRIC INTERVIEW, PSYCHIATRIC HISTORY, AND MENTAL STATUS EXAMINATION

QUESTIONS

Directions: Select the single best response for each of the following questions:

4.1 An interview may be abbreviated if the patient is
   A. Depressed.
   B. Anxious.
   C. Exhibiting psychotic behavior.
   D. All of the above.
   E. None of the above.

4.2 The usual patient-doctor confidentiality is not in force in a psychiatric interview
   A. When the purpose of the examination is to collect information as an expert witness in a court of law.
   B. When the patient is a minor, and information is shared with the parent.
   C. When the purpose of the examination is to advise an employer about the patient's psychiatric fitness.
   D. All of the above.
   E. None of the above; patient-doctor confidentiality is always in force.

4.3 The greatest problem with excessive note taking while taking the history is that
   A. It is difficult to keep the notes organized.
   B. It distracts the patient.
   C. It can inhibit the free exchange of information between the patient and the doctor.

D. It takes too much time during the interview.
E. All of the above.

4.4   Which of the following is **FALSE?**
A. In transference, the patient consciously projects his or her emotions from the past into the psychiatrist-patient relationship.
B. In countertransference, the psychiatrist unconsciously projects his or her emotions from the past onto the patient's personality.
C. A psychiatrist should consult with a colleague when countertransference occurs.
D. All of the above.
E. None of the above.

4.5   Good interviewing technique includes
A. Beginning with close-ended questions at the start of the interview.
B. Referring to the patient by their first name when meeting for the first time in an attempt to establish rapport.
C. Pushing the patient beyond his or her comfort level in terms of expressing feelings.
D. Beginning with potentially charged issues to get them over with.
E. None of the above.

4.6   Incongruity of expressions with verbalizations is common with
A. Anxiety disorders.
B. Psychotic disorders.
C. Depression.
D. Posttraumatic stress disorder.
E. All of the above.

4.7   Errors in interviewing the delusional patient include all of the following **EXCEPT**
A. Quickly reassuring the patient that you understand his or her problem.
B. Focusing the interview on the delusion.
C. Attempting to convince the patient the delusion is not logical.
D. Asking the patient if he or she has acted on the delusion.
E. Agreeing with the patient's delusion.

4.8   A false impression that results from a real stimulus is categorized as
A. Illusion.
B. Hallucination.
C. Derealization.

    D. Depersonalization.

    E. Delusion.

Directions: For each of the statements below, one or more of the answers is correct. Choose

    A. If 1, 2, and 3 are correct.

    B. If only 1 and 3 are correct.

    C. If only 2 and 4 are correct.

    D. If only 4 is correct.

    E. If all are correct.

4.9   During the initial moments of a telephone call by a patient, the psychiatrist should obtain information to determine

    1. The reason for the call.

    2. The location of the patient.

    3. How the caller can be reached.

    4. The urgency of the problem.

4.10   In interviewing elderly patients, it is appropriate to

    1. Slow the pace of the interview.

    2. Review prescribed medications.

    3. Shorten the time of the interview.

    4. Grasp the patient's hand as a sign of reassurance.

4.11   Interviews with the family of a patient

    1. Are necessary for couples therapy.

    2. Should precede the interview with the patient.

    3. Are necessary for a patient in imminent danger.

    4. Involve a free exchange of information about the patient between the psychiatrist and the family.

4.12   The conclusion of the interview should involve

    1. Important areas not yet covered.

    2. Sharing of impressions and a treatment plan by the psychiatrist.

    3. The psychiatrist's request for permission to speak with others and obtain records.

    4. Time for the patient to ask questions.

4.13   Methods of facilitating the interview include

    1. Open-ended questions.

    2. Confrontation about inconsistencies.

        3.   Positive reinforcement.
        4.   False reassurance.

4.14   Obtaining a family history is important in order to obtain information about
        1.   Suicidal attempts or completions.
        2.   Efficacy of medications taken for emotional problems.
        3.   Medical diseases that are common in the family.
        4.   Psychiatric illnesses that are common in the family.

4.15   On the mental status examination, a depressed patient commonly has
        1.   Psychomotor retardation.
        2.   Restricted affect.
        3.   Preoccupation with faults.
        4.   Rapid and loud speech.

ANSWERS

4.1   The answer is **C**. An interview may be abbreviated if the patient is exhibiting psychotic behavior. The interview is typically longer for patients who are depressed or anxious

4.2   The answer is **D**. The usual patient-doctor confidentiality is not in force in a psychiatric interview in such cases as when the purpose of the examination is to collect information as an expert witness in a court of law; when the patient is a minor, and when information is shared with the parent; and when the purpose of the examination is to advise an employer about the patient's psychiatric fitness.

4.3   The answer is **C**. The greatest problem with excessive note-taking is that it can inhibit the free exchange of information between the patient and the doctor.

4.4   The answer is **A**. In transference, the patient unconsciously (not consciously) projects his or her emotions from the past into the psychiatrist-patient relationship.

4.5   The answer is **E**. Good interviewing technique includes beginning with open-ended questions at the start of the interview, referring to the patient by his or her last name when meeting for the first time, not pushing the patient beyond his or her comfort level in terms of expressing feelings, and addressing potentially charged issues later in the interview.

4.6   The answer is **B.** Incongruity of expressions with verbalizations is common with psychotic disorders.

4.7   The answer is **D.** It is important to ask the patient if he or she has acted on the delusion.

4.8   The answer is **A.** A false impression that results from a real stimulus is categorized as an illusion.

4.9   The answer is **E.** The initial moments of a telephone call by a patient requires reason for the call, location of the patient, how the caller can be reached, and a determination of the urgency of the problem.

4.10   The answer is **E.** All of the answers are correct. When one is interviewing elderly patients, it is appropriate to slow the pace of the interview, review prescribed medications, shorten the time of the interview, and grasp the patient's hand as a sign of reassurance.

4.11   The answer is **B.** Interviews with the family of a patient are necessary for couples therapy and for a patient in imminent danger. Generally, they should follow the interview with the patient. Generally, the psychiatrist needs to establish that he or she is not at liberty to share information about the patient with the family.

4.12   The answer is **E.** The conclusion of the interview should involve time for important areas not yet covered, sharing of impressions and a treatment plan by the psychiatrist, the psychiatrist's request for permission to speak with others and obtain records, and time for the patient to ask questions.

4.13   The answer is **B.** Methods of facilitating the interview include open-ended questions and positive reinforcement. Confrontation about inconsistencies and false reassurance tend to obstruct the flow of information.

4.14   The answer is **E.** Obtaining a family history is important in order to obtain information about suicidal attempts or completions, efficacy of medications taken for emotional problems, and medical and psychiatric diseases that are common in the family.

4.15   The answer is **A.** On the mental status examination, a depressed patient commonly has psychomotor retardation, restricted affect, and preoccupation with faults. Speech is usually low volume and monotone.

CHAPTER 5

LABORATORY AND OTHER DIAGNOSTIC TESTS IN PSYCHIATRY

Directions: Select the single best response for each of the following questions:

5.1   An electrocardiogram (ECG) is indicated for
   A.   All patients over 35.
   B.   A patient with a significant cardiac history and who is about to begin an antipsychotic medication.
   C.   A patient beginning a trial of valproic acid.
   D.   A patient beginning a trial of a selective serotonin reuptake inhibitor (SSRI).
   E.   All of the above.

5.2   A blood level of a tricyclic antidepressant is indicated in all of the following situations **EXCEPT**
   A.   Questionable compliance.
   B.   Poor response to the medication at therapeutic doses.
   C.   Populations with sensitivity to side effects (e.g., patients over 60 years of age).
   D.   Severe side effects.
   E.   Side effects that precede a therapeutic response in the first few weeks of therapy.

5.3   The most sensitive and reliable method for evaluating illicit drug abuse is generally considered to be
   A.   High-performance liquid chromatography.
   B.   Gas-liquid chromatography.
   C.   Gas chromatography-mass spectroscopy.

    D. Liquid chromatography-mass spectrometry.

    E. High-performance thin-layer chromatography.

5.4   A computed tomography (CT) scan or magnetic resonance imaging (MRI) is indicated for which of the following indications?

    A. Impaired cognition.

    B. Suspected brain tumor.

    C. First episode of psychosis.

    D. All of the above.

    E. None of the above.

5.5   Which of the following is a common abnormality in patients with schizophrenia as detected by CT?

    A. Decreased ventricular-to-brain ratios.

    B. Decreased occipital lobe mass.

    C. Enlargement of the third ventricle.

    D. All of the above.

    E. None of the above.

5.6   An advantage of functional MRI (fMRI) over positron emission tomography (PET) and single-photon emission computed tomography (SPECT) is

    A. Less exposure to ionizing radiation.

    B. Improved measurement of cortical blood flow in the brain.

    C. Superior spatial/temporal resolution.

    D. A and C.

    E. All of the above.

5.7   How long after initiation of lithium are steady-state blood levels achieved?

    A. 9–12 hours.

    B. 24 hours.

    C. 5 days.

    D. 7 days.

    E. 10 days.

Directions: For each of the statements below, one or more of the answers is correct. Choose

    A. If 1, 2, and 3 are correct.

    B. If only 1 and 3 are correct.

    C. If only 2 and 4 are correct.

    D. If only 4 is correct.

    E. If all are correct.

5.8   Which of the following clues suggest organic mental disorders?

    1. Family history of degenerative brain disease.

    2. History of drug abuse.

    3. Fluctuating mental status.

    4. Abnormal complete blood count (CBC).

5.9   A routine laboratory and diagnostic workup for detecting physical disease in psychiatric patients includes a

    1. CBC.

    2. Thyroid function tests.

    3. Chemistry panel.

    4. Test for syphilis (e.g., VDRL).

5.10   Contraindications for a lumbar puncture include

    1. Use of anticoagulants.

    2. Infection around the site of the puncture.

    3. Increased intracranial pressure.

    4. A history of headache with previous lumbar punctures.

5.11   Advantages of MRI over CT include

    1. Use for patients with a pacemaker.

    2. Better visualization of demyelinating disease.

    3. Less anxiety for the patient during the test.

    4. Better detection of mass lesions.

5.12   Tests to be carried out before lithium initiation include

    1. Pregnancy test in females.

    2. ECG.

    3. Serum creatinine.

    4. Urine culture.

5.13   Side effects of carbamazepine include

    1. Renal dysfunction.

    2. Hepatic dysfunction.

    3. Increased white blood count (WBC).

    4. Hyponatremia.

5.14   PET
      1.   Allows direct visualization of both cortical and subcortical brain function-
           ing.
      2.   Measures cortical blood flow in the brain.
      3.   Measures glucose metabolism in the brain.
      4.   Measures oxygen use by the brain.

ANSWERS

5.1   The answer is **B**. An ECG is indicated for a patient with a significant cardiac
       history and who is about to begin an antipsychotic medication.

5.2   The answer is **E**. A blood level of a tricyclic antidepressant is not indicated when
       side effects precede a therapeutic response in the first few weeks of therapy.

5.3   The answer is **C**. Gas chromatography-mass spectroscopy is generally consid-
       ered to be the most sensitive and reliable method for evaluating illicit drug
       abuse.

5.4   The answer is **D**. A CT scan or MRI is indicated for impaired cognition, sus-
       pected brain tumors, and first episode of psychosis.

5.5   The answer is **C**. Enlargement of the third ventricle is typically seen by CT, as is
       cortical atrophy and increased ventricular-to-brain ratios.

5.6   The answer is **D**. Advantages of fMRI over PET and SPECT are less exposure
       to ionizing radiation and superior spatial/temporal resolution. Measurement
       of cortical blood flow in the brain is not done by fMRI.

5.7   The answer is **C**. Steady-state blood levels are achieved 5 days after initiation of
       lithium.

5.8   The answer is **A**. Clues that suggest organic mental disorders include family
       history of degenerative brain disease, a history of drug abuse, and fluctuating
       mental status.

5.9   The answer is **E**. A routine laboratory and diagnostic workup for detecting
       physical disease in psychiatric patients includes a CBC, thyroid function tests, a
       chemistry panel, and a test for syphilis (e.g., VDRL).

5.10 The answer is **A.** Contraindications for a lumbar puncture include use of anticoagulants, infection around the site of the puncture, and increased intracranial pressure. A history of headache with previous lumbar punctures is not a contraindication. It can often be prevented or minimized by having the patient remain lying down after the procedure.

5.11 The answer is **C.** Advantages of MRI over CT include better visualization of demyelinating disease and better detection of mass lesions. CT, but not MRI, may be used for patients with a pacemaker. CT causes less anxiety for the patient during the test, because 5%–10% of patients are claustrophobic in the MRI apparatus.

5.12 The answer is **A.** Tests (with reasons in parentheses) to be carried out before lithium initiation include pregnancy test in females (teratogenicity), ECG (arrhythmia), and serum creatinine (renal metabolism).

5.13 The answer is **C.** Side effects of carbamazepine include hepatic dysfunction, hyponatremia, and decreased WBC. Of the mood stabilizers, lithium causes decreased renal function and increases the WBC.

5.14 The answer is **E.** PET allows direct visualization of both cortical and subcortical brain functioning and measures cortical blood flow, glucose metabolism, and oxygen use by the brain.

CHAPTER 6

DELIRIUM, DEMENTIA, AND AMNESTIC DISORDERS

Directions: Select the single best response for each of the following questions:

6.1   What percentage of patients with delirium are deceased at 6-month follow-up?
   A. 5%.
   B. 15%.
   C. 25%.
   D. 50%.
   E. 75%.

6.2   A patient is at high risk for delirium if he or she has any of the following predisposing factors **EXCEPT**
   A. AIDS.
   B. Brain damage.
   C. Elderly age.
   D. Drug withdrawal.
   E. Sensory deprivation.

6.3   Which of the following is associated with normal aging according to neuropsychology research?
   A. Increased arousal.
   B. Psychomotor agitation.
   C. Decreased orientation to person.
   D. Diminished performance on nonverbal tasks.
   E. All of the above.

6.4   The most useful screening test for delirium is
   A. Electroencephalogram (EEG).

B. Mini-Mental State Exam (MMSE).
C. Delirium Symptom Interview (DSI).
D. Delirium Rating Scale (DRS).
E. NEECHAM Confusion Scale.

6.5 Which of the following drugs is recommended to treat delirium?
A. Chlorpromazine.
B. Diphenhydramine.
C. Haloperidol.
D. Amitriptyline.
E. Chlorpheniramine.

6.6 The major problem with the MMSE is
A. Its lack of sensitivity (i.e., high rate of false negatives).
B. Its lack of specificity (i.e., high rate of false positives).
C. The time required to complete it is 60 minutes, which is too long for routine use.
D. It cannot be used to follow the patient's clinical course serially.
E. None of the above.

6.7 Which of the following is true?
A. Individuals with dementia of the Alzheimer's type (DAT) are twice as likely to have an affected relative than are control subjects.
B. Patients with familial DAT are more likely to have an early age at onset than are subjects with nonfamilial AD.
C. In early-onset DAT, patients develop the disease before age 40.
D. All of the above.
E. None of the above.

6.8 Delirium occurs in approximately 10%–15% of all hospitalized patients, but at a rate of what percentage in postcardiotomy patients?
A. 10%.
B. 20%.
C. 30%.
D. 40%.
E. 50%.

6.9 The most common cause of amnesia is
A. Neoplasm.
B. Cerebral anoxia.
C. Stroke.

    D. Head trauma.
    E. Epileptic convulsions.

6.10   All of the following are potentially reversible causes of dementia **EXCEPT**
    A. Subdural hematoma.
    B. Normal-pressure hydrocephalus.
    C. Vitamin B_{12} deficiency.
    D. Hypothyroidism.
    E. Parkinson's disease.

Directions: For each of the statements below, one or more of the answers is correct. Choose

    A. If 1, 2, and 3 are correct.
    B. If only 1 and 3 are correct.
    C. If only 2 and 4 are correct.
    D. If only 4 is correct.
    E. If all are correct.

6.11   Patients with dementia syndrome of depression (DSD)
    1. Have more severe sleep disturbance, particularly early morning awakening, than patients with primary dementia.
    2. Have symptoms resembling cortical dementia rather than subcortical dementia.
    3. More frequently report a history of previous affective disorder than patients with primary dementia.
    4. Respond best to a combination of antidepressants and cholinesterase inhibitors.

6.12   Drugs that can cause delirium include
    1. Naproxen.
    2. Levodopa.
    3. Lithium.
    4. Cimetidine.

6.13   Vascular dementia usually can be distinguished from dementia of the Alzheimer's type by
    1. The occurrence of hallucinations.
    2. Abnormal speech melody.
    3. The prevalence of delusions.
    4. Abrupt onset.

6.14   Clinical features of delirium usually include
    1.   Decreased attention.
    2.   Disturbance in the sleep-wake cycle.
    3.   An acute onset or a fluctuating course.
    4.   Disorientation to person.

6.15   Routine labs for the evaluation of delirium include
    1.   Blood chemistries.
    2.   Drug levels.
    3.   Blood count.
    4.   Urinalysis.

6.16   Behavioral disturbances in a patient with dementia should be routinely managed with
    1.   Benzodiazepines.
    2.   Antihistamines.
    3.   Dopamine agonists.
    4.   Behavioral interventions.

6.17   Which of the following are true about delirium and the EEG?
    1.   Slowing of brain rhythms can be seen on the EEG.
    2.   Abnormalities on the EEG are correlated with deficiencies in the patient's ability to draw a clock.
    3.   Spectral EEG analysis is more useful than standard EEG techniques, particularly in agitated patients.
    4.   High-voltage fast activity can be seen on the EEG in patients with delirium tremens.

6.18   Diseases causing subcortical dementia include
    1.   Parkinson's disease.
    2.   Human immunodeficiency virus (HIV).
    3.   Huntington's disease.
    4.   Pick's disease.

6.19   The management of delirium always includes
    1.   Benzodiazepines for control of agitation.
    2.   Placement of the patient near the nursing station.
    3.   Antihistamines for insomnia.
    4.   Regular monitoring of vital signs.

6.20 Familial DAT
    1. Accounts for 50% of cases of DAT.
    2. Is more likely to have an early onset than nonfamilial DAT.
    3. Can be detected before onset of symptoms by routine laboratory evaluation.
    4. May be associated with abnormalities on chromosome 21.

ANSWERS

6.1 The answer is **C.** Twenty-five percent of patients are deceased at 6-month follow-up.

6.2 The answer is **E.** Patients are not at high risk for delirium if they only have a sensory deprivation experience.

6.3 The answer is **D.** Diminished performance on nonverbal tasks is associated with normal aging according to neuropsychology research. Other findings include decreased arousal, psychomotor slowing, and forgetfulness of nonverbal information.

6.4 The answer is **B.** The MMSE is the most useful screening test for delirium.

6.5 The answer is **C.** Haloperidol is recommended to treat delirium.

6.6 The answer is **A.** The major problem with the MMSE is its lack of sensitivity (i.e., high rate of false negatives).

6.7 The answer is **B.** Patients with familial DAT are more likely to have an early age at onset.

6.8 The answer is **D.** The rate of delirium in postcardiotomy patients is approximately 30%.

6.9 The answer is **D.** The most common cause of amnesia is head trauma.

6.10 The answer is **E.** Dementia due to Parkinson's disease is not reversible. Reversible causes of dementia include subdural hematoma, normal-pressure hydrocephalus, vitamin B_{12} deficiency, and hypothyroidism.

6.11   The answer is **B.** Patients with DSD have more severe sleep disturbance (particularly early morning awakening) and more frequently report a history of previous affective disorder than patients with primary dementia. Their symptoms typically resemble subcortical dementia rather than cortical dementia. They respond best to antidepressants, and cholinesterase inhibitors are not indicated.

6.12   The answer is **E.** Naproxen, levodopa, lithium, and cimetidine can cause delirium.

6.13   The answer is **C.** Vascular dementia usually can be distinguished from DAT by abnormal speech melody and abrupt onset.

6.14   The answer is **C.** Clinical features of delirium usually include decreased attention and an acute onset or a fluctuating course. Disturbance in the sleep-wake cycle commonly occurs, but not in all patients. Patients are rarely disoriented to person.

6.15   The answer is **E.** Routine labs for the evaluation of delirium include blood chemistries, blood count, drug levels, and urinalysis.

6.16   The answer is **D.** Behavioral disturbances in a patient with dementia should be routinely managed with behavioral interventions in addition to an antipsychotic medication. Benzodiazepines, antihistamines, and dopamine agonists cause significant worsening of the patient's behavioral problems.

6.17   The answer is **A.** In patients with delirium, the electroencephalogram (EEG) often shows slowing of brain rhythms. Abnormalities on the EEG are correlated with deficiencies in the patient's ability to draw a clock. Spectral EEG analysis is more useful than standard EEG techniques, particularly in agitated patients. *Low-voltage*, not high-voltage, fast activity can be seen on the EEG in patients with delirium tremens.

6.18   The answer is **A.** Diseases causing subcortical dementia include Parkinson's disease, human immunodeficiency virus (HIV), and Huntington's disease. Pick's disease causes a fronto-temporal cortical dementia.

6.19   The answer is **C.** The management of delirium always includes placement of the patient near the nursing station and regular monitoring of vital signs. Antihistamines for insomnia may worsen the patient's condition. Benzodiazepines are indicated for the etiology of sedative-hypnotic withdrawal. They are also sometimes used in combination with antipsychotic medication for management of agitation.

6.20   The answer is **C.** Familial dementia of the Alzheimer's type (DAT) is more
        likely to have an early onset than nonfamilial DAT and may be associated with
        abnormalities on chromosome 21. It accounts for only 5% of cases of DAT. It
        cannot be detected by routine laboratory evaluation.

CHAPTER 7

ALCOHOL AND OTHER PSYCHOACTIVE SUBSTANCE USE DISORDERS

QUESTIONS

Directions: Select the single best response for each of the following questions:

7.1   The lifetime prevalence of alcohol abuse is approximately
   A. 2%.
   B. 5%.
   C. 10%.
   D. 20%.
   E. 30%.

7.2   The most common comorbid disorders for women with alcoholism are
   A.   Other substance abuse disorders.
   B.   Psychotic disorders.
   C.   Personality disorders.
   D.   Anxiety disorders.
   E.   Dissociative disorders.

7.3   Alcoholics commit suicide at rates similar to patients with
   A.   Anxiety disorders.
   B.   Depression.
   C.   Eating disorders.
   D.   Dissociative disorders.
   E.   Dementia.

7.4   The preferred treatment for a patient with hallucinations from alcohol withdrawal is
        A. Benzodiazepines.
        B. Brief, supportive counseling.
        C. Talking the patient down from the hallucinations.
        D. Antipsychotic medication.
        E. Behavioral therapy with strict limit setting.

7.5   Naltrexone for management of alcohol disorders
        A. Is used for acute alcohol withdrawal.
        B. Is used for 3 months and then discontinued, with its effects lasting long term.
        C. Reduces the number of drinking days during the maintenance phase of alcohol abstinence.
        D. May cause liver damage.
        E. Produces a toxic reaction like Antabuse if alcohol is used concurrently.

7.6   For the purpose of detoxification, the maintenance dose of benzodiazepine is best estimated by
        A. History.
        B. Physical examination.
        C. The pentobarbital challenge test.
        D. A and C.
        E. All of the above.

7.7   After using cannabinoids, a patient will test positive via urine samples for up to
        A. 12–24 hours.
        B. 1–7 days.
        C. 8–10 days.
        D. 14 days.
        E. 21 days.

7.8   Death rates for patients with opioid dependence are increased by what rate over nondependent patients
        A. 10-fold.
        B. 20-fold.
        C. 30-fold.
        D. 40-fold.
        E. 50-fold.

7.9　A common side effect of methadone is
　　A. Agitation.
　　B. Increased libido.
　　C. Ankle edema.
　　D. Diarrhea.
　　E. Headache.

7.10　In comparison to methadone, L-Alphacetylmethadol (LAAM) has
　　A. A shorter half-life.
　　B. Increased mood side effects.
　　C. A quicker onset of action.
　　D. Better rates of retention of patients in treatment programs.
　　E. All of the above.

7.11　Which of the following have been found to be effective in the treatment of cocaine abuse and dependence?
　　A. Drug urine tests.
　　B. Interpersonal therapy.
　　C. Behavior therapy.
　　D. All of the above.
　　E. None of the above.

7.12　Antipsychotics are **NOT** the drug of choice for hallucinations secondary to phencyclidine because
　　A. Higher rates of extrapyramidal side effects occur in these patients.
　　B. The hallucinations spontaneously resolve within hours.
　　C. The antipsychotics may cause anticholinergic psychosis.
　　D. The antipsychotics are not effective.
　　E. None of the above.

Directions: For each of the statements below, one or more of the answers is correct. Choose

　　A. If 1, 2, and 3 are correct.
　　B. If only 1 and 3 are correct.
　　C. If only 2 and 4 are correct.
　　D. If only 4 is correct.
　　E. If all are correct.

7.13   Substance dependence (SD) differs from substance abuse (SA) in that
1.   In SD, the same substance is taken to relieve or avoid withdrawal symptoms.
2.   In SD, the substance is taken in larger amounts or over a longer time than was intended.
3.   In SD, a great deal of time is spent in activities necessary to obtain the substance, use the substance, or recover from its effects.
4.   In SD, the substance is continued despite knowledge of having had a persistent or recurrent physical or psychological problem from the substance.

7.14   Self-administered screening tests for alcoholism include the
1.   Michigan Alcoholism Screening Test (MAST).
2.   Addiction Severity Index (ASI).
3.   Alcohol Use Disorders Identification Test (AUDIT).
4.   Minnesota Multiphasic Personality Inventory (MMPI).

7.15   Which of the following behaviors meet the DSM-IV criteria for substance abuse?
1.   Repeated absences from work due to substance use.
2.   Repeated arrests for drunk driving.
3.   Repeated arguments with spouse about drinking behavior.
4.   Chronic depression.

7.16   Which of the following laboratory findings is associated with alcohol abuse?
1.   Elevated serum γ-glutamyltransferase (GGT).
2.   Elevated albumin.
3.   Elevated mean corpuscular volume (MCV).
4.   Increased white cell count.

7.17   Medical complications of alcoholism include
1.   Hypothyroidism.
2.   Trauma.
3.   Rheumatoid arthritis.
4.   Cancer.

7.18   Seizures from alcohol withdrawal
1.   Generally occur at 72 hours after the last drink.
2.   Are associated with hyperglycemia.
3.   Are associated with respiratory acidosis.
4.   Are associated with hypomagnesemia.

7.19 Delirium tremens
1. Involves visual but not auditory hallucinations.
2. May last 4–5 weeks.
3. Have a mortality rate of 25% even when treated.
4. Usually develop 2–4 days after the last drink.

7.20 Psychosocial interventions for alcoholism include
1. Warnings by the physician about using alcohol.
2. Psychoeducation.
3. Family counseling.
4. Group therapy.

7.21 In narcotic-addicted patients, disorders that are commonly comorbid include
1. Depression.
2. Personality disorders.
3. Antisocial disorders.
4. Eating disorders.

7.22 A significant side effect of clonidine, which is used for opioid detoxification, is
1. Headache.
2. Sedation.
3. Diarrhea.
4. Hypotension.

7.23 The effects of cocaine include
1. Hyperalertness.
2. Grandiosity.
3. Visual and tactile hallucinations.
4. Irritability.

7.24 Urine drug testing may be positive seven days after use for which of the following drugs?
1. Amphetamines.
2. Phencyclidine.
3. Lysergic acid diethylamide (LSD).
4. Marijuana.

7.25 Which of the following pharmacologic treatments are efficacious for smoking cessation?
1. Naltrexone.
2. Bupropion (Zyban).

3. Benzodiazepines.
4. Nicotine patch.

ANSWERS

7.1   The answer is **C.** The lifetime prevalence of alcohol abuse is about 10% (9.4%).

7.2   The answer is **D.** The most common comorbid disorders for women with alcoholism are anxiety disorders.

7.3   The answer is **D.** Alcoholics commit suicide at rates similar to patients with depression.

7.4   The answer is **A.** The treatment of choice for a patient with hallucinations from alcohol withdrawal is benzodiazepines.

7.5   The answer is **C.** Naltrexone for management of alcohol disorders reduces craving and the number of drinking days during the maintenance phase of alcohol abstinence. It is not used for acute alcohol withdrawal. Its effects do not appear to last after it is discontinued. It does not cause liver damage. It does not produce a toxic reaction (like Antabuse) if alcohol is used concurrently.

7.6   The answer is **D.** For the purpose of detoxification, the maintenance dose of benzodiazepine is best estimated by the history and pentobarbital challenge test.

7.7   The answer is **B.** After using cannabinoids, a patient will test positive via urine samples for up to 1–7 days.

7.8   The answer is **B.** Death rates for patients with opioid dependence are increased by 20-fold over nondependent patients because of infection, homicide, suicide, overdose, and AIDS.

7.9   The answer is **C.** A common side effect of methadone is ankle edema. Other side effects include sedation, decreased libido, and constipation.

7.10   The answer is **B.** In comparison to methadone, L-alphacetylmethadol (LAAM) has increased mood side effects. It has a longer half-life, a slower onset on action, and reduced rates of retention of patients in treatment programs.

7.11   The answer is **D.** Drug urine tests, interpersonal therapy, and behavior therapy have been found to be effective in the treatment of cocaine abuse and dependence.

7.12   The answer is **C.** Antipsychotics are not the drug of choice for hallucinations secondary to phencyclidine because the antipsychotics may cause anticholinergic psychosis. Benzodiazepines are the drug of choice for phencyclidine intoxication.

7.13   The answer is **A.** SD differs from SA in that in SD, the same substance is taken to relieve or avoid withdrawal symptoms, the substance is taken in larger amounts or over a longer time than was intended, and a great deal of time is spent in activities necessary to obtain the substance, use the substance, or recover from its effects. However, in *both* SD and SA, the substance is continued despite knowledge of having had a persistent or recurrent physical or psychological problem from the substance.

7.14   The answer is **B.** Self-administered screening tests for alcoholism include the MAST and the AUDIT. The ASI must be administered by trained staff. The MMPI is not a screening test used to detect alcohol use.

7.15   The answer is **A.** Behaviors that meet the DSM-IV criteria for substance abuse include repeated absences from work due to substance use, repeated arrests for drunk driving, and repeated arguments with spouse about drinking behavior.

7.16   The answer is **B.** Laboratory findings associated with alcohol abuse include elevated serum GGT and elevated MCV.

7.17   The answer is **C.** Medical complications of alcoholism include trauma and cancer (e.g., oral).

7.18   The answer is **D.** Seizures from alcohol withdrawal are associated with hypomagnesemia. They generally occur 7–36 hours after the last drink, and are associated with hypoglycemia and respiratory alkalosis.

7.19   The answer is **C.** DTs usually develop 2–4 days after the last drink and may last 4–5 weeks. DTs may involve visual, auditory, and tactile hallucinations and have a mortality rate of 1% when treated.

7.20   The answer is **E.** Psychosocial interventions for alcoholism include warnings by the physician about using alcohol, psychoeducation, family counseling, and group therapy.

7.21   The answer is **A.** In narcotic-addicted patients, disorders that are commonly comorbid include depression, personality disorders, and antisocial disorders.

7.22   The answer is **C.** Significant side effects of clonidine, which is used for opioid detoxification, are sedation and hypotension.

7.23   The answer is **E.** The effects of cocaine include hyperalertness, grandiosity, visual and tactile hallucinations, and irritability.

7.24   The answer is **C.** Urine drug testing may be positive 7 days after use of phencyclidine and marijuana.

7.25   The answer is **C.** Bupropion (Zyban) and the nicotine patch are efficacious pharmacologic treatments for smoking cessation.

CHAPTER 8

SCHIZOPHRENIA, SCHIZOPHRENIFORM DISORDER, AND DELUSIONAL (PARANOID) DISORDERS

Directions: Select the single best response for each of the following questions:

8.1   If a patient with bipolar disorder or major depression were misdiagnosed with schizophrenia, the patient would
      A.   Be deprived of the most appropriate treatment available.
      B.   Condemned to an unnecessarily chronic course of illness.
      C.   Potentially suffer permanent and irreversible medication side effects.
      D.   All of the above.
      E.   None of the above.

8.2   Paranoid type of schizophrenia is associated with a (an)
      A.   Earlier age at onset.
      B.   Worse outcome.
      C.   Better premorbid functioning.
      D.   Greater likelihood of divorce.
      E.   Family history of obsessive-compulsive disorder.

8.3   In the Iowa 500 study, evaluation of the patients years later revealed that
      A.   10% had committed suicide.
      B.   25% had never married.
      C.   50% were in mental institutions.
      D.   90% had never worked.
      E.   All of the above.

8.4   Which of the following features is associated with a favorable outcome in schizophrenia?
        A.   Presence of obsessive symptoms.
        B.   Normal neurological examination.
        C.   An insidious onset of symptoms.
        D.   A clear sensorium on mental status examination.
        E.   Absence of affective symptoms.

8.5   Which of the following is true about schizophrenia?
        A.   Approximately 90% of females have an onset of schizophrenia by age 30.
        B.   Approximately 40% of males have an onset of schizophrenia after age 35.
        C.   A sibling of a schizophrenic patient has about a 10% chance of developing schizophrenia.
        D.   A child of a schizophrenic patient has an increased risk for developing schizophrenia, but not schizotypal personality disorder.
        E.   None of the above.

8.6   Increased mortality in schizophrenic patients is primarily due to
        A.   Cancer.
        B.   Malnutrition.
        C.   Immunodeficiency.
        D.   Underutilization of medical services.
        E.   Suicide and accidents.

8.7   Ventricular enlargement on structural imaging of schizophrenia patients is associated with
        A.   Positive symptoms.
        B.   Negative symptoms.
        C.   Good response to treatment.
        D.   Lack of assaultive behavior.
        E.   History of head trauma.

8.8   Which of the following medications is considered a first-line treatment for schizophrenia?
        A.   Risperidone.
        B.   Haloperidol.
        C.   Olanzapine.
        D.   A and B.
        E.   All of the above.

8.9   Which of the following is true about maintenance medication for schizophrenia?
   A.   Once the acute episode is in remission, maintenance medication is needed for approximately 6 months.
   B.   Lower doses may be used but the patient is at higher risk for relapse at these doses than those used for the acute phase.
   C.   If it is decided that maintenance medication is no longer needed, it may be discontinued at once.
   D.   A reliable dose-response curve has been established for each medication during the maintenance phase.
   E.   Depot forms of administration do not yield higher rates of compliance than oral forms of administration.

8.10   A patient who moves frequently because she says her neighbors are conspiring to rob her, and who is unable to keep a steady job because she always comes to believe that her co-workers are plotting against her, most likely would be diagnosed with
   A.   Persecutory-type delusional disorder.
   B.   Capgras' syndrome.
   C.   Shared psychotic disorder.
   D.   Paranoid schizophrenia.
   E.   Paranoid disorder.

8.11   Patients with schizophrenia are hospitalized less than in the past because of
   A.   Family interventions.
   B.   The increased effectiveness of higher doses of antipsychotic medication.
   C.   The advent of day treatment programs.
   D.   A and C only.
   E.   All of the above.

8.12   Delusional disorder is characterized by
   A.   An onset between 20 and 40 years of age.
   B.   Bizarre delusions lasting at least 1 month.
   C.   Functioning that is not markedly impaired aside from the delusion.
   D.   Paranoid, disorganized, catatonic, and undifferentiated types.
   E.   A and C only.

Directions: For each of the statements below, one or more of the answers is correct. Choose

   A.   If 1, 2, and 3 are correct.
   B.   If only 1 and 3 are correct.

C. If only 2 and 4 are correct.

D. If only 4 is correct.

E. If all are correct.

8.13   The differential diagnosis of schizophrenia includes the following medical illnesses

1. Acute intermittent porphyria.
2. Vitamin B_{12} deficiency.
3. Systemic lupus erythematous.
4. Lyme disease.

8.14   Schneider's first-rank symptoms include

1. Auditory hallucinations.
2. Thought broadcasting.
3. Thought insertion.
4. Formal thought disorder.

8.15   Which of the following factors is associated with a good outcome for schizophrenic patients?

1. Short duration of psychotic episode.
2. Marriage.
3. High social class.
4. Acute onset of illness.

8.16   Neurobiological studies have shown that many of the symptoms of schizophrenia

1. Are consistent with temporolimbic disease.
2. May be caused by a gene on chromosome 5.
3. May be caused by frontal lobe dysfunction.
4. May be exacerbated by family environment.

8.17   Negative symptoms in a patient with schizophrenia may be

1. Caused by antipsychotic medication.
2. An intrinsic part of the illness.
3. Difficult to discern from a depression.
4. An indicator of good prognosis.

8.18   Disorganized (hebephrenic) schizophrenia is associated with

1. Poor long-term prognosis.
2. Affective flattening.
3. Early onset of the disorder.
4. Avolition.

8.19   Schizophreniform patients may be eventually diagnosed with
   1.   Schizophrenia.
   2.   Bipolar disorder.
   3.   Schizoaffective disorder.
   4.   Major depressive disorder with psychosis.

8.20   The prodromal phase for a schizophrenic patient is characterized by
   1.   Auditory hallucinations.
   2.   A duration of months to years.
   3.   Increased productivity.
   4.   Social withdrawal.

8.21   Features associated with a negative outcome for schizophrenia include
   1.   Family history of schizophrenia.
   2.   Low socioeconomic class.
   3.   Chronic duration of symptoms.
   4.   Female gender.

8.22   Contemporary theories explain schizophrenia as a consequence of
   1.   A defect in monitoring others' behavior.
   2.   A disruption of circuits connecting the forebrain and thalamus.
   3.   Increased prepulse inhibition.
   4.   Abnormalities in programmed cell death (apoptosis).

8.23   Which of the following does **NOT** support the dopamine hypothesis of schizophrenia?
   1.   Dopamine agonists increase symptoms.
   2. D_2 receptors are prominent in the striatum but not the limbic system.
   3.   Dopamine antagonists decrease symptoms.
   4.   Postmortem brain analysis reveals an increase of D_2 receptors in the caudate and nucleus accumbens.

8.24   Which of the following facilitates adherence to medication?
   1.   Lowering the dose to reduce side effects.
   2.   Psychoeducation.
   3.   Prescribing an atypical antipsychotic medication.
   4.   Case management.

8.25   Psychosocial rehabilitation for patients with schizophrenia includes
   1.   Having the patient involved with the development and implementation of his or her rehabilitation program.

    2.   Finding the patient a job.

    3.   Finding appropriate and affordable housing.

    4.   Providing funding for family trips.

ANSWERS

8.1   The answer is **D.** The patient would be deprived of the most appropriate treatment available (e.g., antidepressant or mood stabilizer). The patient would be condemned to an unnecessarily chronic course of illness instead of the appropriate intermittent course of a mood disorder. If the patient was given typical antipsychotic medication long term, he or she may suffer permanent and irreversible medication side effects.

8.2   The answer is **C.** Paranoid type of schizophrenia is associated with *better* premorbid functioning, a *later* age at onset, a *better* outcome, and a *reduced* likelihood of divorce. Family history of obsessive-compulsive disorder is not associated with paranoid type.

8.3   The answer is **A.** In the Iowa 500 study, evaluation of the patients years later revealed that 10% had committed suicide, 67% had never married, 18% were in mental institutions, and 58% had never worked.

8.4   The answer is **B.** Normal neurological examination is associated with a favorable outcome in schizophrenia. The presence of obsessive symptoms, an insidious onset of symptoms, (ironically) a clear sensorium on mental status examination, and an absence of affective symptoms are associated with a negative prognosis.

8.5   The answer is **C.** A sibling of a schizophrenic patient has about a 10% chance of developing schizophrenia. Approximately 67% of females have an onset of schizophrenia by age 30. Approximately 2% of males have an onset of schizophrenia after age 35. A child of a schizophrenic patient has an increased risk for developing schizophrenia and schizotypal personality disorder.

8.6   The answer is **E.** Increased mortality in schizophrenic patients is primarily due to suicide and accidents.

8.7   The answer is **B.** Ventricular enlargement on structural imaging of schizophrenia patients is associated with negative symptoms.

8.8 The answer is **E**. Risperidone, haloperidol, and olanzapine are considered first-line treatments for schizophrenia

8.9 The answer is **B**. Lower doses may be used but the patient is at higher risk for relapse at these doses than those used for the acute phase. Once the acute episode is in remission, maintenance medication is needed for at least 1–2 years and perhaps permanently. If it is decided that maintenance medication is no longer needed, it should be discontinued over weeks to months. Reliable dose-response curves have not yet been established for medications during the maintenance phase. Depot forms of administration yield higher rates of compliance than oral forms of administration.

8.10 The answer is **A**. A patient who moves frequently because she says her neighbors are conspiring to rob her, and who is unable to keep a steady job because she always comes to believe that her co-workers are plotting against her, most likely would be diagnosed with persecutory-type delusional disorder.

8.11 The answer is **D**. Patients with schizophrenia are hospitalized less than in the past because of family interventions and the advent of day treatment programs. Higher doses of antipsychotic medication are not necessarily more effective.

8.12 The answer is **C**. Delusional disorder is characterized by functioning that is not markedly impaired aside from the delusion. The onset is typically between 35 and 55 years of age with *non*bizarre delusions lasting at least 1 month. Types of delusional disorders include erotomanic, grandiose, jealous, persecutory, somatic, and mixed.

8.13 The answer is **A**. The differential diagnosis of schizophrenia includes acute intermittent porphyria, vitamin B_{12} deficiency, and systemic lupus erythematous. Lyme disease causes depressive and anxiety symptoms but not psychotic symptoms.

8.14 The answer is **A**. Schneider's first-rank symptoms include thought broadcasting, thought insertion, and auditory hallucinations. Formal thought disorder is not a first-rank delusion or symptom.

8.15 The answer is **E**. Factors that predict a good outcome for schizophrenic patients include short duration of psychotic episode, married, high social class, and acute onset of illness.

8.16   The answer is **B.** Neurobiological studies have shown that many of the symptoms of schizophrenia are consistent with temporolimbic disease and may be caused by frontal lobe dysfunction. Genetic molecular techniques are being used to investigate the existence of a schizophrenia gene; family studies focus on family environment. No clear chromosomal etiology has been found.

8.17   The answer is **A.** Negative symptoms in a patient with schizophrenia may be caused by antipsychotic medication, an intrinsic part of the illness, and difficult to discern from a depression. Negative symptoms are generally an indicator of poor prognosis.

8.18   The answer is **E.** Disorganized (hebephrenic) schizophrenia is associated with a poor long-term prognosis, affective flattening, an early onset of the disorder, and avolition.

8.19   The answer is **B.** Schizophreniform patients may eventually be diagnosed with schizophrenia, bipolar disorder, schizoaffective disorder, or major depression with psychosis.

8.20   The answer is **C.** The prodromal phase for a schizophrenic patient is characterized by duration of months to years, social withdrawal, and *decreased* productivity. Auditory hallucinations occur in the acute phase.

8.21   The answer is **A.** Features associated with a negative outcome for schizophrenia include a family history of schizophrenia, low socioeconomic class, a chronic duration of symptoms, and male (not female) gender.

8.22   The answer is **C.** Contemporary theories explain schizophrenia as a consequence of a defect in self-monitoring (not monitoring others' behavior), a disruption of circuits connecting the forebrain and thalamus, *decreased* prepulse inhibition, and abnormalities in programmed cell death (apoptosis).

8.23   The answer is **C.** D_2 receptors are prominent in the striatum but not the limbic system and yet the limbic system is the presumed target for neuroleptic drug action. Postmortem brain analysis reveals an increase of D_2 receptors in the caudate and nucleus accumbens that may be an artifact of antipsychotic treatment rather than a reflection of the disorder itself.

8.24   The answer is **E.** Lowering the dose to reduce side effects, psychoeducation, prescribing an atypical antipsychotic medication, and case management all enhance adherence to medication.

8.25   The answer is **B**. The patient should be involved with the development and implementation of his or her rehabilitation program and appropriate and affordable housing should be located. The patient receives job training in preparation for a job, but a job may be overwhelming. The family is involved with the rehabilitation but does not receive money for activities.

CHAPTER 9
MOOD DISORDERS

QUESTIONS

Directions: Select the single best response for each of the following questions:

9.1 What percentage of patients with major depressive disorders (MDD) eventually commit suicide?
  A. 10%.
  B. 15%.
  C. 20%.
  D. 25%.
  E. More than 25%.

9.2 In comparison to unipolar depression, which of the following statements about bipolar depression is **FALSE?**
  A. Bipolar depression has an earlier onset.
  B. Bipolar depression has more psychomotor agitation.
  C. Bipolar depression has more insomnia.
  D. Bipolar depression has a greater risk of suicide.
  E. None of the above.

9.3 Major depressive disorder
  A. May include depressive episodes with or without manic episodes.
  B. Requires that a patient have a depressed mood.
  C. Is caused by a medical disorder by definition.
  D. Is usually a recurrent disorder.
  E. All of the above.

9.4 Which of the following statements about MDD and dysthymic disorder (DD) is **FALSE?**
  A. MDD causes significantly more impairment in work, leisure activities, relationships, and general health than DD.

      B. Comorbid conditions are approximately the same for MDD and DD.

      C. MDD requires a depressed mood or a loss of interest or pleasure, whereas DD requires a depressed mood.

      D. More symptoms are required to diagnose MDD than DD.

      E. MDD and DD respond to the same antidepressant regimens.

9.5   Psychosis associated with MDD

      A. Occurs in 60%–75% of patients with MDD.

      B. Usually involves hallucinations without delusions.

      C. May include auditory, visual, or olfactory hallucinations.

      D. Usually occurs with the first depressive episode.

      E. All of the above.

9.6   Risk factors for the rapid cycling type of bipolar disorder include all of the following **EXCEPT**

      A. Female gender.

      B. Bipolar I disorder.

      C. Hypothyroidism.

      D. Use of alcohol and stimulants.

      E. Mental retardation.

9.7   The essential feature of bipolar I disorder is

      A. One or more episodes of major depression before the first manic episode.

      B. A pattern of depression-mania-euthymia.

      C. A pattern of mania-depression-euthymia.

      D. A history of at least one manic episode.

      E. Hypomania and recurrent major depressive episodes without mania.

9.8   Which of the following is true about mood disorders?

      A. Unipolar depression is most likely to recur in the fall.

      B. Bipolar depression is most likely to recur in the fall.

      C. Seasonal depression usually begins in the month of January.

      D. Symptoms of seasonal depression usually last 1–2 months.

      E. All of the above.

9.9   Medications known to cause depression include

      A. Diltiazem.

      B. Clonazepam.

      C. Levodopa.

      D. Captopril.

      E. All of the above.

9.10 Patients suffering from acute depression also are often diagnosed with a personality disorder. In a study that assessed patients after successful treatment for depression
   A. Identical rates of personality disorder were diagnosed.
   B. Personality disorders were diagnosed 50% less often.
   C. Cluster A diagnoses were most commonly comorbid with depression.
   D. The presence of a personality disorder was a predictor of good prognosis.
   E. None of the above.

9.11 Lithium
   A. Is dosed to achieve a blood level range of 50–100 mg/mL.
   B. Is the mood stabilizer of choice for rapid cycling type of bipolar disorder.
   C. Is not discontinued rapidly (unless the patient is toxic) because of increased risk of bipolar mania relapse.
   D. Commonly causes tardive dyskinesia.
   E. None of the above.

9.12 In the treatment of bipolar mania, benzodiazepines
   A. Are indicated for the management of agitation.
   B. Reduce the amount of antipsychotic medication when given concurrently.
   C. Facilitate sleep.
   D. Have been noted to contribute to neurotoxicity when used concurrently with lithium.
   E. All of the above.

9.13 Which treatment is as effective as bright lights for seasonal affective disorder?
   A. Cognitive therapy.
   B. Fluoxetine.
   C. Electroconvulsive therapy (ECT).
   D. Venlafaxine.
   E. None of the above.

Directions: For each of the statements below, one or more of the answers is correct. Choose

   A. If 1, 2, and 3 are correct.
   B. If only 1 and 3 are correct.
   C. If only 2 and 4 are correct.
   D. If only 4 is correct.
   E. If all are correct.

9.14   Diagnostic criteria for a major depressive episode include
   1.   Depressed mood that is worse only in the morning.
   2.   Insomnia or hypersomnia.
   3.   Inability to set aside worries in more than one area of life experience.
   4.   Excessive or inappropriate guilt.

9.15   Factors suggesting an increased risk of suicide include
   1.   Active substance abuse.
   2.   Family history of seasonal affective disorder.
   3.   History of suicide attempts.
   4.   Female sex.

9.16   Common symptoms of seasonal depression include
   1.   Depressed mood.
   2.   Increased appetite and weight.
   3.   Daytime drowsiness.
   4.   Suicidal ideation.

9.17   The prevalence of depression in the following medical disorders is approximately
   1.   10%–30% with breast cancer.
   2.   10%–75% with cerebrovascular accidents.
   3.   50% with Alzheimer's disease.
   4.   10%–25% with colon cancer.

9.18   Changes in sleep architecture for patients with depression include
   1.   Decreased sleep continuity.
   2.   Increased time in rapid eye movement (REM) sleep.
   3.   Decreased REM latency.
   4.   Difficulty entering and remaining in slow-wave sleep.

9.19   A common finding on neuroimaging of patients with depression is
   1.   Cortical atrophy.
   2.   Increased size of the caudate nucleus.
   3.   Subcortical white matter hyperintensities.
   4.   Enlarged lateral ventricles.

9.20   The following factors have been found to increase the risk of relapse and recurrence of unipolar depression
   1.   Inadequate treatment.
   2.   Psychosis.

3. Discontinuation of effective treatment.
4. Medical etiologies.

9.21 Common side effects of tricyclic antidepressants include
1. Constipation.
2. Sexual dysfunction.
3. Orthostatic hypotension.
4. Agitation.

9.22 Which of the following drugs commonly causes sexual dysfunction?
1. Fluoxetine.
2. Sertraline.
3. Paroxetine.
4. Bupropion.

9.23 Standard treatments for bipolar disorder include
1. A mood stabilizer.
2. ECT.
3. Psychoeducation.
4. Cognitive therapy.

9.24 Behavior therapy for depression
1. Targets behaviors such as self-blame and negativism.
2. Rewards behaviors such as problem solving.
3. Does not usually use educational approaches.
4. Uses guided practice and homework assignments.

9.25 Clues to the presence of bipolarity in a patient with depression include
1. Delusions.
2. Highly recurrent depression.
3. Family history of depression.
4. Mood-incongruent psychotic symptoms.

ANSWERS

9.1 The answer is **B.** Fifteen percent of patients with MDD eventually commit suicide.

9.2 The answer is **B.** In comparison to unipolar depression, bipolar depression has *less* psychomotor agitation. Bipolar depression also has an earlier onset, more insomnia, and a greater risk of suicide.

9.3   The answer is **D**. MDD is usually a recurrent disorder. A patient may not have manic episodes in addition to depressive episodes. A patient must have either depressed mood or loss of interest or pleasure. MDD is restricted to mood episodes not caused by a medical disorder or substance disorders.

9.4   The answer is **A**. MDD and DD cause equal impairment in work, leisure activities, relationships, and general health. Comorbid conditions are approximately the same for MDD and DD. MDD requires a depressed mood or a loss of interest or pleasure, whereas DD requires a depressed mood. More symptoms are required to diagnose MDD (5) than DD (3). MDD and DD respond to the same antidepressant regimens.

9.5   The answer is **C**. Psychosis associated with major depressive disorder may include auditory, visual, or olfactory hallucinations. It occurs in 16%–54% of patients with MDD. Hallucinations without delusions occur in only 3%–25% of patients. The psychosis usually occurs after several depressive episodes without psychosis.

9.6   The answer is **B**. Risk factors for the rapid cycling type of bipolar disorder include bipolar II (not I) disorder, female gender, hypothyroidism, use of alcohol and stimulants, and mental retardation.

9.7   The answer is **D**. The essential feature of bipolar I disorder is a history of at least one manic episode.

9.8   The answer is **B**. Bipolar depression is most likely to recur in the fall. Unipolar depression is more likely to recur in the spring. Seasonal depression usually begins in the month of November and symptoms usually last 5–6 months.

9.9   The answer is **E**. Medications known to cause depression include diltiazem, clonazepam, levodopa, and captopril.

9.10   The answer is **B**. After successful treatment for depression, personality disorders were diagnosed 50% less frequently. Cluster B diagnoses are most commonly comorbid with depression. Presence of a personality disorder comorbid with depression is a potential negative predictor of poor prognosis.

9.11   The answer is **C**. Lithium is not discontinued rapidly (unless the patient is toxic) because of increased risk of bipolar mania relapse. It is dosed to achieve a blood level range of 0.8–1.2 meq/mL. Anticonvulsants are the mood stabilizers of choice for rapid cycling type of bipolar disorder. Lithium does not cause tardive dyskinesia.

9.12   The answer is **E.** In the treatment of bipolar mania, benzodiazepines are indicated for the management of agitation, reduce the amount of antipsychotic medication when given concurrently, facilitate sleep, and have been noted to contribute to neurotoxicity when used concurrently with lithium.

9.13   The answer is **B.** Fluoxetine is as effective as bright lights for seasonal affective disorder.

9.14   The answer is **C.** Diagnostic criteria for a major depressive episode include insomnia or hypersomnia, and excessive or inappropriate guilt. The depressed mood may be worse in the morning or evening. Inability to set aside worries in more than one area of life experience is a criteria for general anxiety disorder.

9.15   The answer is **B.** Factors suggesting an increased risk of suicide include active substance abuse and history of suicide attempts. Family history of seasonal affective disorder has not been evaluated in terms of risk of suicide. Male (not female) sex increases risk.

9.16   The answer is **A.** Common symptoms of seasonal depression include depressed mood, increased appetite and weight, and daytime drowsiness. Suicidal ideation is uncommon but may occur.

9.17   The answer is **E.** The prevalence of depression is 10%–30% with breast cancer, 10%–75% with cerebrovascular accidents, 50% with Alzheimer's disease, and 10%–25% with colon cancer.

9.18   The answer is **E.** Changes in sleep architecture for patients with depression include decreased sleep continuity, increased time in REM sleep, decreased REM latency, and difficulty entering and remaining in slow-wave sleep.

9.19   The answer is **D.** A common finding on neuroimaging of patients with depression is enlarged lateral ventricles.

9.20   The answer is **E.** Inadequate treatment, psychosis, discontinuation of effective treatment, and medical etiologies have been found to increase the risk of relapse and recurrence of unipolar depression.

9.21   The answer is **A.** Common side effects of tricyclic antidepressants include constipation, sexual dysfunction, and orthostatic hypotension. Agitation occurs rarely.

9.22   The answer is **A.** Selective serotonin reuptake inhibitors (fluoxetine, sertraline, and paroxetine) cause a significant amount of sexual dysfunction, which is rare with bupropion.

9.23   The answer is **A.** Standard treatments for bipolar disorder include a mood stabilizer, ECT, and psychoeducation. The efficacy of cognitive therapy has not been assessed for bipolar disorder.

9.24   The answer is **C.** Behavior therapy for depression rewards behaviors such as problem solving and uses educational approaches, guided practice, and homework assignments. *Cognitive* therapy does not target behaviors such as self-blame and negativism.

9.25   The answer is **C.** Clues to the presence of bipolarity in a patient with depression include highly recurrent depression and mood-incongruent psychotic features.

CHAPTER 10
ANXIETY DISORDERS

QUESTIONS

Directions: Select the single best response for each of the following questions:

10.1 A patient's first panic attack may be precipitated by
A. A life-threatening illness.
B. Loss of a close friend.
C. Giving birth to a child.
D. Use of a mind-altering drug (e.g., marijuana).
E. All of the above.

10.2 According to the catecholamine theory, panic disorder is caused by
A. Abnormal receptor function leading to decreased inhibitory activity.
B. Massive β-adrenergic nervous system discharge.
C. Increased discharge of central nervous system noradrenergic nuclei.
D. Aberrant metabolic changes induced by lactate infusion.
E. None of the above.

10.3 Which of the following is true?
A. Panic disorder is not more frequent among patients with mitral valve prolapse than it is among the general population.
B. Hypoglycemia can cause panic disorder.
C. Panic disorder is distinguished from generalized anxiety disorder in that the onset of the former is always precipitated by a trauma.
D. All of the above.
E. None of the above.

10.4 The treatment of choice for agoraphobia is
A. Reassurance.
B. Psychoeducation.
C. Supportive psychotherapy.

D. Cognitive-behavior therapy.

E. An antidepressant.

10.5 General anxiety disorder may be distinguished from major depression by

A. A greater frequency of initial than middle or late insomnia.

B. A lack of diurnal mood fluctuation.

C. A lack of anhedonia.

D. All of the above.

E. None of the above.

10.6 The most extensively studied pharmacological treatment for obsessive-compulsive disorder (OCD) is

A. Sertraline.

B. Desipramine.

C. Clomipramine.

D. Clonazepam.

E. Buspirone.

10.7 In social phobia, the patient's central fear is that he or she

A. Will make a mistake.

B. Will be criticized.

C. Will embarrass him- or herself.

D. Will embarrass another person.

E. None of the above.

10.8 Social phobia

A. Has an onset usually in the teenage and early adult years.

B. Has a significant genetic component to its etiology.

C. Has a course that improves with old age.

D. Does not typically respond to treatment with monoamine oxidase inhibitors (MAOIs).

E. All of the above.

10.9 The treatment of choice for specific phobia is

A. Reassurance.

B. Psychoeducation.

C. Graded exposure.

D. Cognitive therapy.

E. An antidepressant.

10.10 The most common compulsion that patients experience in OCD is
   A. Avoiding.
   B. Checking.
   C. Repeating.
   D. Striving for completeness.
   E. Washing.

10.11 A therapeutic response to medication for patients with obsessive-compulsive disorder means symptom reduction by what percentage?
   A. 10%–20%.
   B. 30%–40%.
   C. 50%–60%.
   D. 70%–80%.
   E. 90%–100%.

Directions: For each of the statements below, one or more of the answers is correct. Choose

   A. If 1, 2, and 3 are correct.
   B. If only 1 and 3 are correct.
   C. If only 2 and 4 are correct.
   D. If only 4 is correct.
   E. If all are correct.

10.12 Panic attacks can occur in
   1. Panic disorder with agoraphobia.
   2. Social phobia.
   3. Panic disorder without agoraphobia.
   4. Posttraumatic stress disorder.

10.13 The lactate panicogenic metabolic theory is based on studies that show
   1. Lactate provocation produces attacks that closely resemble regular attacks.
   2. Attacks per lactate provocation are blocked by drugs that block regular attacks.
   3. Transient intracerebral hypercapnia may induce attacks and occurs upon lactate provocation.
   4. Lactate provocation induces metabolic alkalosis.

10.14 A weakness inherent in the learning theory model of phobias is
   1. The theory only applies to panic attacks resulting from the same stimulus.
   2. Many phobias do not begin with a trauma in which the phobic object is associated with an unpleasant unconditioned stimulus.

    3.   The range of phobic objects is too broad to classify.

    4.   The theory does not account for the maintenance of phobic symptoms.

10.15 Predictors of poor outcome with panic disorder include

    1.   Comorbid major depression.

    2.   Greater severity of initial attacks.

    3.   Separation from a parent by death or divorce.

    4.   An anxious-fearful personality style.

10.16 Which of the following are true for both panic disorder and general anxiety disorder?

    1.   The course improves with old age.

    2.   They are commonly comorbid with depression.

    3.   The suicide rate parallels that of depression.

    4.   They are more common in females.

10.17 An antidepressant trial for panic disorder may require concurrent benzodiazepine therapy during the first 4–8 weeks in order to

    1.   Reduce the amount of intervening anticipatory anxiety.

    2.   Reduce the frequency of panic attacks.

    3.   Reduce the agitation or "jittery" feeling patients have starting the antidepressant.

    4.   Reduce the likelihood of sexual side effects from the antidepressant.

10.18 Buspirone

    1.   Is an effective treatment for panic disorder.

    2.   Is an effective treatment for general anxiety disorder.

    3.   Works within 1–2 weeks.

    4.   Has a better side effect profile than benzodiazepines.

10.19 Which of the following anxiety disorders are more common in women than in men?

    1.   General anxiety disorder.

    2.   Social phobia.

    3.   Panic disorder.

    4.   Specific phobia.

10.20 Psychological defenses common to patients with OCD include

    1.   Projection.

    2.   Isolation of affect.

3. Denial.
4. Undoing.

10.21 Which of the following findings are true about OCD and medical disorders?
1. OCD may occur after head trauma.
2. A high incidence of neurological premorbid illness in OCD.
3. OCD patients often have abnormalities on the EEG and auditory evoked potentials.
4. An association of OCD with diabetes mellitus.

10.22 Patients with posttraumatic stress disorder reexperience the trauma through
1. Recurrent and intrusive recollections.
2. Recurrent dreams.
3. Physiological reactivity on exposure to external cues of the trauma.
4. Hallucinations of the trauma.

10.23 Risk factors for developing posttraumatic stress disorder after traumatic exposure include
1. Poor parental attachments.
2. History of anxiety disorders.
3. History of family anxiety disorders.
4. History of seizure disorders.

10.24 Treatment of posttraumatic stress disorder includes
1. Behavior therapy.
2. Carbamazepine.
3. Brief dynamic psychotherapy.
4. Selective serotonin reuptake inhibitors (SSRIs).

10.25 Parameters for the therapist doing brief dynamic therapy for veterans with posttraumatic stress disorder include
1. Initial rapport building.
2. Limit-setting and supportive confrontation.
3. Maintaining a positive treatment attitude.
4. Defocusing on stress and focusing on current life events.

ANSWERS

10.1 The answer is **E**. A patient's first panic attack may be precipitated by a life-threatening illness, the loss of a close friend, giving birth to a child, or the use of a mind-altering drug (e.g., marijuana).

10.2   The answer is **B.** According to the catecholamine theory, panic disorder is caused by massive β-adrenergic nervous system discharge.

10.3   The answer is **A.** Panic disorder is not more frequent among patients with mitral valve prolapse than it is among the general population. Although many patients believe their panic disorder is caused by hypoglycemia, this condition is *not* known to cause any psychiatric disorder. For many patients with panic disorder, no precipitating trauma can be identified.

10.4   The answer is **D.** Cognitive-behavior therapy is the treatment of choice for agoraphobia.

10.5   The answer is **D.** General anxiety disorder may be distinguished from major depression by a greater frequency of initial than middle or late insomnia, a lack of diurnal mood fluctuation, and a lack of anhedonia.

10.6   The answer is **C.** The most extensively studied pharmacological treatment for OCD is clomipramine.

10.7   The answer is **C.** In social phobia, the patient's central fear is that they will act in a way that they will embarrass themselves.

10.8   The answer is **A.** The onset of social phobia is usually in the teenage and early adult years. It does not have a significant genetic component to its etiology. The course of social phobia is quite chronic. Patients with social phobia typically respond to MAOIs.

10.9   The answer is **C.** The treatment of choice for specific phobia is graded exposure.

10.10   The answer is **E.** The most common compulsion that patients experience in OCD is washing.

10.11   The answer is **C.** A therapeutic response to medication for patients with OCD means symptom reduction by 50%–60%.

10.12   The answer is **E.** Panic attacks occur in panic disorder with or without agoraphobia, social phobia, and posttraumatic stress disorder, as well as other anxiety disorders.

10.13 The answer is **E.** The lactate panicogenic metabolic theory is based on studies that show that lactate provocation produces attacks that closely resemble regular attacks and are blocked by drugs that block regular attacks. Transient intracerebral hypercapnia may induce attacks and occurs upon lactate provocation, as does metabolic alkalosis.

10.14 The answer is **C.** Weaknesses inherent in the learning theory model of phobias include the fact that many phobias do not begin with a trauma in which the phobic object is associated with an unpleasant unconditioned stimulus and, in addition, that the theory does not account for the maintenance of phobic symptoms.

10.15 The answer is **E.** Predictors of poor outcome with panic disorder include comorbid major depression, greater severity of initial attacks, separation from a parent by death or divorce, and an anxious-fearful personality style.

10.16 The answer is **C.** Both panic disorder and general anxiety disorder are commonly comorbid with depression and more common in females. The course for panic disorder improves with old age, but this is not so for general anxiety disorder. Only the suicide rate for panic disorder parallels that of depression.

10.17 The answer is **A.** An antidepressant trial for panic disorder may require concurrent benzodiazepine therapy during the first 4–8 weeks in order to reduce the amount of intervening anticipatory anxiety, and the agitation or "jittery" feeling patients have starting the antidepressant. Benzodiazepines may also reduce the frequency of panic attacks.

10.18 The answer is **C.** Buspirone is an effective treatment for general anxiety disorder, but not for panic disorder. It works within 3–4 weeks and has a better side effect profile than benzodiazepines.

10.19 The answer is **E.** General anxiety disorder, social phobia, panic disorder, and specific phobia are more common in women than men.

10.20 The answer is **C.** Defenses common to patients with OCD include isolation of affect and undoing.

10.21 The answer is **A.** Patients may suffer from OCD after head trauma. Patients who develop OCD have a high incidence of premorbid neurological illness. OCD patients often have EEG and auditory evoked potential abnormalities. OCD is associated with diabetes insipidus, not mellitus.

10.22   The answer is **E.** Patients with posttraumatic stress disorder reexperience the trauma through recurrent and intrusive recollections, recurrent dreams, physiological reactivity on exposure to external cues of the trauma, and hallucinations of the trauma.

10.23   The answer is **A.** Risk factors for developing posttraumatic stress disorder after traumatic exposure include poor parental attachments, history of anxiety disorders, and history of family anxiety disorders.

10.24   The answer is **E.** Treatment for posttraumatic stress disorder includes behavior therapy, carbamazepine, brief dynamic psychotherapy, and SSRIs.

10.25   The answer is **E.** Parameters for the therapist doing brief dynamic therapy for veterans with posttraumatic stress disorder include initial rapport building, limit setting and supportive confrontation, maintaining a positive treatment attitude, and defocusing on stress and focusing on current life events.

CHAPTER 11
SOMATOFORM DISORDERS

QUESTIONS

Directions: Select the single best response for each of the following questions:

11.1   One of the classic psychosomatic illnesses described by Alexander is
   A.   Hypothyroidism.
   B.   Peptic ulcer.
   C.   Irritable bowel syndrome.
   D.   Multiple sclerosis.
   E.   Migraine headache.

11.2   What percentage of patients with body dysmorphic disorder never marry?
   A.   10%.
   B.   25%.
   C.   50%.
   D.   75%.
   E.   90%.

11.3   According to DSM-IV, a diagnosis of somatization disorder requires
   A.   3 symptoms.
   B.   8 symptoms.
   C.   13 symptoms.
   D.   18 symptoms.
   E.   23 symptoms.

11.4   Standard treatment of somatization disorder includes
   A.   Antidepressants.
   B.   Anxiolytics.
   C.   Repeated batteries of labs.
   D.   Development of a therapeutic alliance.
   E.   None of the above. The condition is not treatable.

11.5   According to the diagnostic criteria for somatization disorder, the sexual or re-
       productive symptom may be
       A. Erectile dysfunction.
       B. Irregular menses.
       C. Excessive menstrual bleeding.
       D. Vomiting throughout pregnancy.
       E. All of the above.

11.6   Which of the following is true?
       A. In conversion disorder, symptoms are not intentionally produced.
       B. Symptoms of blindness, aphonia, and paralysis are associated with a good
           prognosis for conversion disorder patients.
       C. The term *conversion* derives from conversion of psychological conflict into
           somatic symptoms.
       D. All of the above.
       E. None of the above.

11.7   Many patients with conversion disorder
       A. Have comorbid somatization disorder.
       B. Are later correctly diagnosed with a neurological illness that explain their
           symptoms.
       C. Respond well to selective SSRIs.
       D. Require psychiatric hospitalization.
       E. All of the above.

11.8   Which of the following is the essential feature of hypochondriasis?
       A. Deficits affecting voluntary motor or sensory function.
       B. Exaggerated symptoms.
       C. History of physical complaints not explained by a known medical condi-
           tion.
       D. Fear of having a serious illness.
       E. None of the above.

Directions: For each of the statements below, one or more of the answers is correct.
Choose

       A. If 1, 2, and 3 are correct.
       B. If only 1 and 3 are correct.
       C. If only 2 and 4 are correct.
       D. If only 4 is correct.
       E. If all are correct.

11.9 Which of the following is important in distinguishing somatization disorder from medical illness?
1. Absence of characteristic laboratories of the suggested medical disorder.
2. Onset of symptoms at an age considered young for the suggested medical illness.
3. Involvement of multiple organ systems.
4. Concurrent depressive and/or anxiety symptoms.

11.10 Which of the following is important in distinguishing somatization disorder from an anxiety disorder?
1. Sexual and menstrual problems.
2. Histrionic personality traits.
3. Conversion and dissociative symptoms.
4. Presence of substance abuse.

11.11 A frequent and important complication of somatization disorder is
1. Repeated surgical operations.
2. Drug dependence.
3. Suicide attempts.
4. Marital separation or divorce.

11.12 The most reliable predictor that a patient with conversion disorder will not later be diagnosed with a physical disorder is
1. The symptom deficit is a voluntary sensory function.
2. A history of major depression.
3. Long duration of the symptom.
4. A history of previous conversion or other unexplained symptoms.

11.13 Routine treatment of somatization disorder includes
1. Regularly scheduled appointments.
2. Selective serotonin reuptake inhibitors (SSRIs).
3. Psychoeducation.
4. Long-term psychodynamic psychotherapy.

11.14 Somatization disorder may be associated with
1. Antisocial personality disorder.
2. Borderline personality disorder.
3. Alcoholism.
4. Frontal lobe dysfunction.

11.15 Conversion disorder may be treated by
    1. Direct confrontation about the hypothesized conflict.
    2. Hypnotic therapy.
    3. A trial of anticonvulsants.
    4. Narcoanalysis.

11.16 Management of hypochondriasis should include the following treatments:
    1. Regular visits that are not based on the evaluation of symptoms.
    2. SSRIs.
    3. Focus of visits from symptoms to social or interpersonal problems.
    4. Benzodiazepines.

11.17 Which of the following symptoms make body dysmorphic disorder unlikely?
    1. Preoccupation with body shape and size.
    2. A sense of inappropriateness of one's primary and secondary sex characteristics.
    3. A general perceived unattractive appearance in association with poor self-esteem.
    4. Bizarre delusions and hallucinations.

11.18 Treatments found to be efficacious for body dysmorphic disorder include
    1. Long-term psychotherapy.
    2. Benzodiazepines.
    3. Surgery.
    4. SSRIs.

11.19 The treatment of pseudocyesis should emphasize
    1. Empathic education that the patient is not pregnant.
    2. An ultrasound to demonstrate the patient is not pregnant.
    3. Exploration as to why the patient "needs" to be pregnant.
    4. Computed tomography (CT) and/or magnetic resonance imaging (MRI) of the abdomen to demonstrate the patient is not pregnant.

11.20 Which of the following are true about somatization disorder?
    1. It is equally common in males and females.
    2. Men tend to report fewer symptoms than women.
    3. The lifetime risk for somatization disorder is approximately 10%.
    4. Patients report fewer symptoms to nonphysicians than physicians.

ANSWERS

11.1   The answer is **B**. The classic psychosomatic illnesses described by Alexander are peptic ulcer, thyrotoxicosis, asthma, rheumatoid arthritis, neurodermatitis, and hypertension.

11.2   The answer is **D**. Seventy-five percent of patients with body dysmorphic disorder never marry.

11.3   The answer is **B**. According to DSM-IV, a diagnosis of somatization disorder requires eight symptoms.

11.4   The answer is **D**. Standard treatment of somatization disorder includes the development of a firm therapeutic alliance.

11.5   The answer is **E**. According to the diagnostic criteria for somatization disorder, the sexual or reproductive symptom may be erectile dysfunction, irregular menses, excessive menstrual bleeding, or vomiting throughout pregnancy.

11.6   The answer is **D**. All of the statements are true.

11.7   The answer is **B**. Many patients with conversion disorder are later correctly diagnosed with a neurological illness that explains their symptoms.

11.8   The answer is **D**. The essential feature of hypochondriasis is fear of having a serious illness.

11.9   The answer is **E**. Findings that distinguish somatization disorder from medical illness are absence of characteristic laboratories of the suggested medical illness, early onset of symptoms at an age considered young for the suggested medical illness, involvement of multiple organ systems, and concurrent depressive and/or anxiety symptoms.

11.10 The answer is **A**. Sexual and menstrual problems, histrionic personality traits, and conversion and dissociative symptoms are important in distinguishing somatization disorder from an anxiety disorder. Substance disorder occurs commonly with somatization and anxiety disorders.

11.11 The answer is **E**. Frequent and important complications of somatization disorder include repeated surgical operations, drug dependence, suicide attempts, and marital separation or divorce.

11.12　The answer is **D.** The most reliable predictor that a patient with conversion disorder will not later be diagnosed with a physical disorder is a history of previous conversion or other unexplained symptoms.

11.13　The answer is **B.** Routine treatment of somatization disorder includes regularly scheduled appointments and psychoeducation. SSRIs are used only if the patient has a depression or anxiety disorder. The efficacy of long-term psychodynamic psychotherapy is unknown for somatization disorder.

11.14　The answer is **E.** Somatization disorder may be associated with antisocial personality disorder, borderline personality disorder, alcoholism, and frontal lobe dysfunction.

11.15　The answer is **C.** Conversion disorder may be treated by hypnotic therapy and narcoanalysis.

11.16　The answer is **B.** Management of hypochondriasis should include the following treatments: regular visits that are not based on the evaluation of symptoms and shifting the focus of visits from symptoms to social or interpersonal problems. SSRIs are used only if the patient has a comorbid depressive or anxiety disorder.

11.17　The answer is **E.** Preoccupation with body shape and size suggests anorexia. A sense of inappropriateness of one's primary and secondary sex characteristics suggests a sexual disorder. A general perceived unattractive appearance in association with poor self-esteem suggests depression or a personality disorder. Bizarre delusions and hallucinations suggest a psychotic disorder.

11.18　The answer is **D.** SSRIs have been found to be efficacious for body dysmorphic disorder.

11.19　The answer is **A.** The treatment of pseudocyesis should emphasize empathic education that the patient is not pregnant, an ultrasound to demonstrate the patient is not pregnant, and an exploration as to why the patient "needs" to be pregnant. CT and MRI are costly and unnecessary in light of the availability of ultrasound.

11.20　The answer is **C.** The disorder is much more common in females than males. Men tend to report fewer symptoms than women and patients report fewer symptoms to nonphysicians than physicians. The lifetime risk for somatization disorder is approximately 2%.

CHAPTER 12

FACTITIOUS DISORDERS AND MALINGERING

QUESTIONS

Directions: Select the single best response for each of the following questions:

12.1 Most patients with factitious disorders
   A. Have jobs in the field of business.
   B. Have multisystem complaints.
   C. Are middle-aged men.
   D. Are young women.
   E. None of the above.

12.2 The primary explanation precipitating factitious symptoms is
   A. Sexual abuse.
   B. Childhood illness.
   C. Parental abuse.
   D. Poor self-image.
   E. Fear of abandonment.

12.3 Management of factitious disorder in the medical hospital includes
   A. Removing the patient from the hospital as soon as the diagnosis is made.
   B. Directly confronting the patient about the deception.
   C. Interventions by the psychiatrist rather than the medical team.
   D. Initiation of a selective serotonin reuptake inhibitor (SSRI).
   E. Examination of the medical teams' concerns and beliefs about the patient.

12.4 Diagnostic criteria for factitious disorder by proxy (Munchausen syndrome by proxy) specify that
   A. The proxy has motivation to make the child suffer.
   B. The proxy has external incentives (e.g., economic gain).

C. The proxy has to be the mother.
D. All of the above.
E. None of the above.

12.5   The treatment of choice for factitious disorder by proxy is
A. Cognitive therapy.
B. Pharmacotherapy.
C. Long-term psychotherapy.
D. Long-term hospitalization.
E. None of the above.

12.6   Patients suspected of malingering
A. Usually are later diagnosed with a previously unknown medical disorder.
B. Commonly have comorbid dissociative disorders.
C. May eventually be correctly diagnosed with a severe psychiatric disorder (e.g., schizophrenia).
D. Are as willing as Munchausen patients to have invasive procedures performed.
E. All of the above.

12.7   Warning signs of malingering include all of the following **EXCEPT**
A. Symptoms are vague, ill defined, and do not conform to discrete diagnostic entities.
B. Injuries do not appear to be self-inflicted.
C. There is a history of recurrent injuries or accidents.
D. There is a concomitant diagnosis of antisocial personality disorder.
E. The patient requests addicting on commonly abused drugs to treat the disorder.

12.8   To evaluate a patient suspected of malingering,
A. Use one's subjective confidence or intuition as the guide to diagnosis.
B. Rely solely on information from the interview, physical examination, and laboratory examination.
C. Order extensive laboratory tests to rule out medical disorders.
D. Perform serial evaluations to check for consistency of responses.
E. All of the above.

Directions: For each of the statements below, one or more of the answers is correct. Choose

A. If 1, 2, and 3 are correct.
B. If only 1 and 3 are correct.

C. If only 2 and 4 are correct.
D. If only 4 is correct.
E. If all are correct.

12.9 Malingering should be suspected when which of the following is present or takes place?
1. Lack of cooperation during diagnostic evaluation.
2. Ill-defined symptoms.
3. Referral of the patient to the physician by an attorney.
4. 12 month duration of symptoms.

12.10 Factors suggesting a factitious disorder include
1. A course that is atypical for a medical disorder.
2. Acceptance without concerns of invasive diagnostic procedures.
3. Failure to respond as expected to usual therapies.
4. History of antisocial personality disorder.

12.11 Potential explanations for factitious disorders include
1. Disturbed parental relationships.
2. Histories of early or extended hospitalizations.
3. Physical or sexual abuse.
4. Trauma leading to excessive use of psychological defenses including dissociation, denial, and projection.

12.12 Warning signs for factitious disorder by proxy include
1. The child's signs and symptoms abate or do not occur when the child is separated from the parent.
2. Another child in the family has had unexplained illness or death.
3. The parent has taken the child to numerous medical providers, resulting in multiple diagnostic evaluations but neither cure nor definitive diagnosis has occurred.
4. The other parent is closely involved.

12.13 Disorders that are commonly comorbid with factitious disorders include
1. Mood disorders.
2. Substance disorders.
3. Eating disorders.
4. Anxiety disorders.

12.14 Which of the following disorders involves the intentional feigning of symptoms?
1. Factitious disorders.
2. Conversion disorders.
3. Malingering.
4. Somatoform disorders.

12.15 Which of the following are true about Munchausen's syndrome?
1. It comprises about 10% of factitious disorder patients.
2. It is characterized by pseudologia fantastica.
3. Patients have dramatic and life-threatening presentations.
4. It usually refers to factitious disorder patients with physical rather than psychological symptoms.

ANSWERS

12.1   The answer is **D.** Most patients with factitious disorders are young women. Many have health-related jobs and single-system complaints.

12.2   The answer is **E.** The primary explanation precipitating factitious symptoms is fear of abandonment.

12.3   The answer is **E.** Management of factitious disorder includes examination of the medical teams' concerns and beliefs (countertransference) about the patient. A meeting is helpful to determine the setting for ongoing treatment before the patient leaves the hospital. Indirect confrontation or none at all are standard approaches. A collaborative effort between *all* staff (not just psychiatric staff) is indicated. An SSRI is not indicated unless a comorbid condition requires it.

12.4   The answer is **E.** Diagnostic criteria for factitious disorder by proxy specify that the motivation of the proxy is to assume the sick role by proxy. The proxy does not have external incentives (e.g., economic gain). The proxy is usually the mother but can be any important, primary caregiver.

12.5   The answer is **C.** The treatment of choice for factitious disorder by proxy is long-term psychotherapy.

12.6   The answer is **C.** Malingerers may eventually be correctly diagnosed with a severe psychiatric disorder (e.g., schizophrenia).

12.7   The answer is **B**. One warning sign of malingering is that injuries appear to be self-inflicted, rather than not self-inflicted.

12.8   The answer is **D**. To evaluate suspected malingering, perform serial evaluations to check for consistency of responses. Do not use one's subjective confidence or intuition as the guide to diagnosis. Obtain information from the interview, physical examination, laboratory examination, and collateral sources.

12.9   The answer is **A**. Malingering should be suspected when a patient does not co-operate during the diagnostic evaluation, presents with ill-defined symptoms, and was referred to the physician by an attorney. Symptoms of malingering patients are usually much shorter than 12 months in duration.

12.10   The answer is **A**. Factors suggesting a factitious disorder include a course that is atypical for the medical disorder, acceptance without concerns of invasive diagnostic procedures, and a failure to respond as expected to usual therapies. Antisocial personality disorder may be associated with malingering but is not associated with factitious disorders.

12.11   The answer is **E**. Potential explanations for factitious disorders include disturbed parental relationships, histories of early or extended hospitalizations, physical or sexual abuse, and trauma leading to excessive use of psychological defenses including dissociation, denial, and projection.

12.12   The answer is **A**. Warning signs for factitious disorder by proxy include signs and symptoms abate or do not occur when the child is separated from the parent, another child in the family has had unexplained illness or death, and the parent has taken the child to numerous medical providers, resulting in multiple diagnostic evaluations but neither cure nor definitive diagnosis. The other parent is noticeably *not* involved.

12.13   The answer is **A**. Disorders commonly comorbid with factitious disorders include mood, substance, and eating disorders.

12.14   The answer is **B**. Factitious disorders and malingering involve the intentional feigning of symptoms. Conversion and somatoform disorders do not involve intentional feigning of symptoms.

12.15   The answer is **E**. Munchausen's syndrome comprises about 10% of factitious disorder patients, is characterized by pseudologia fantastica, and patients have dramatic and life-threatening presentations. It usually refers to factitious disorder patients with physical rather than psychological symptoms.

CHAPTER 13
DISSOCIATIVE DISORDERS

QUESTIONS

Directions: Select the single best response for each of the following questions:

13.1   According to most studies, what percentage of those who experience serious trauma will later become symptomatic?
A.   5%.
B.   10%.
C.   25%.
D.   50%.
E.   75%.

13.2   The most common of all dissociative disorders is
A.   Dissociative amnesia.
B.   Dissociative fugue.
C.   Dissociative identity disorder.
D.   Depersonalization disorder.
E.   Dissociative trance disorder.

13.3   The most important treatment for a patient with dissociative fugue is
A.   Directly confronting the patient about reality.
B.   Observation, since the disorder usually remits on its own.
C.   Clear limit setting to reduce problematic behavior.
D.   Helping the patient work through interpersonal or intrapsychic issues that underlie dissociative defenses.
E.   All of the above.

13.4   Which of the following statements about dissociative identity disorder (DID) is **FALSE?**
A.   Patients are symptomatic for approximately 6 years before diagnosis.
B.   It is the most common dissociative disorder.

C. Its overall prevalence in North America is approximately 0.1%–1%.
D. It usually emerges between adolescence and the third decade of life.
E. Untreated, it is a recurrent and chronic disorder.

13.5 Pharmacologic treatments for dissociative identity disorder
A. Help to manage comorbid conditions rather than the disorder itself.
B. Reduce dissociative episodes.
C. Are not tolerated, generally, because of these patients' propensity to have side effects.
D. A and C.
E. None of the above.

13.6 Secrets between identities in a patient with dissociative identity disorder are best managed by
A. Hospitalization.
B. A trial with selective serotonin reuptake inhibitor (SSRI).
C. Hypnosis.
D. Educating the identities and securing a commitment from each identity that information will be shared among them.
E. Behavior therapy with adversive reinforcement for those who keep secrets.

Directions: For each of the statements below, one or more of the answers is correct. Choose

A. If 1, 2, and 3 are correct.
B. If only 1 and 3 are correct.
C. If only 2 and 4 are correct.
D. If only 4 is correct.
E. If all are correct.

13.7 Repression is characterized by
1. Information being kept out of consciousness because of a variety of experiences, fears, or wishes over time.
2. Information storage in a discrete and untransformed manner.
3. Information stored in an archeological manner, at various depths, and hence not equally accessible.
4. Information that usually can be retrieved by a single trial of hypnosis.

13.8 Dissociative disorders are most common in patients with
1. Dysthymia.
2. Borderline personality disorder.

3. Anorexia nervosa.
4. A history of physical or sexual abuse.

13.9 Dissociative fugue involves
1. Sudden, unexpected, purposeful travel away from home.
2. Loss of identity or assumption of a new identity.
3. Inability to recall important details of one's past.
4. An alternating pattern between the old and new identities.

13.10 Depersonalization disorder may remit in response to
1. No treatment.
2. Cognitive therapy.
3. Self-hypnosis.
4. Systematic desensitization.

13.11 Common comorbid illnesses of dissociative identity disorder are
1. Substance abuse and dependence disorders.
2. Anxiety disorders.
3. Depressive disorders.
4. Psychotic disorders.

13.12 Trance states
1. Have a duration of less than one hour.
2. Result in fatigue at the termination of the trance.
3. Are episodic with normal behavior between trances.
4. Are more common in patients with low social class and poor educational levels.

ANSWERS

13.1 The answer is **C**. According to most studies, 25% of those who experience serious trauma will later become symptomatic.

13.2 The answer is **A**. The most common of all dissociative disorders is dissociative amnesia.

13.3 The answer is **D**. The most important treatment for a patient with dissociative fugue is helping the patient work through interpersonal or intrapsychic issues that underlie dissociative defenses.

13.4   The answer is **B.** Dissociative identity disorder is not the most common dissociative disorder.

13.5   The answer is **A.** Pharmacologic treatments for dissociative identity disorder help to manage comorbid conditions rather than the disorder itself.

13.6   The answer is **D.** Secrets between identities in a patient with dissociative identity disorder are best managed by educating the identities and securing a commitment from each identity that information will be shared among them.

13.7   The answer is **B.** Repression is characterized by information being kept out of consciousness because of a variety of experiences, fears, or wishes over time. It is stored in an archeological manner, at various depths, and hence not equally accessible. The information is stored in a disguised and fragmented manner. It usually can be retrieved by repeated trials of questioning, therapy, or analysis.

13.8   The answer is **C.** Dissociative disorders are most common in patients with Axis II disorders and a history of physical or sexual abuse.

13.9   The answer is **A.** Dissociative fugue involves sudden, unsuspected, purposeful travel away from home; loss of identity or assumption of a new identity; and inability to recall important details of one's past. The old and new identities do not alternate, in contrast with dissociative identity disorder.

13.10   The answer is **B.** Depersonalization disorder may remit in response to no treatment or self-hypnosis.

13.11   The answer is **B.** Common comorbid illnesses of dissociative identity disorder are the substance disorders and depressive disorders.

13.12   The answer is **E.** Trance states have a duration of less than 1 hour, result in fatigue at the termination of the trance, are episodic with normal behavior between trances, and are more common in patients with low social class and poor educational skills.

CHAPTER 14

SEXUAL AND GENDER IDENTITY DISORDERS

QUESTIONS

Directions: Select the single best response for each of the following questions:

14.1   Patients with borderline personality disorder have transient wishes to change gender because of their
    A.   Mood lability.
    B.   Fear of abandonment.
    C.   Identity diffusion.
    D.   Chronic suicidal ideation.
    E.   All of the above.

14.2   Gender identity is established
    A.   At birth.
    B.   At 3 months of age.
    C.   At 3 years of age.
    D.   At 6 years of age.
    E.   At puberty.

14.3   Which of the following medications can interfere with sexual functioning?
    A.   Tricyclic antidepressants.
    B.   Monoamine oxidase inhibitors.
    C.   Selective serotonin reuptake inhibitors.
    D.   Antipsychotic medications.
    E.   All of the above.

14.4   The incidence of gender identity disorder of childhood is
    A.   5%.
    B.   10%.

    C. 15%.

    D. 20%.

    E. Unknown.

14.5   The treatment of gender identity disorder for a boy includes

    A. Helping the boy avoid ostracism and humiliation.

    B. Increasing the boy's comfort with his own sex.

    C. Developing a close, trusting relationship between a male therapist and the boy.

    D. Stopping parental encouragement of feminine behaviors.

    E. All of the above.

14.6   All of the following drugs or medications cause sexual dysfunction **EXCEPT**

    A. Alcohol.

    B. Cocaine.

    C. Propranolol (Inderal), which is a β blocker.

    D. Bupropion (Wellbutrin).

    E. Chlorpromazine (Thorazine).

14.7   The excitement stage in the sexual cycle is characterized by

    A. An increase in heart rate and blood pressure.

    B. Sexual fantasies.

    C. Erotic feelings that lead to vaginal lubrication in women and penile erection in men.

    D. A desire to be sexual.

    E. A and C.

14.8   The prevalence of premature ejaculation for males in the general population is approximately

    A. 5%.

    B. 15%.

    C. 25%.

    D. 35%.

    E. 45%.

14.9   The primary treatment for a sexual aversion disorder is

    A. Psychoeducation.

    B. Cognitive therapy.

    C. Systematic desensitization.

    D. Psychodynamic psychotherapy.

    E. Biofeedback.

14.10 The first step and most likely way for a woman with general anorgasmia to become orgasmic is
A. Sensate focus exercises.
B. Cognitive therapy.
C. Systematic desensitization.
D. A program of directed masturbation.
E. A medication trial.

Directions: For each of the statements below, one or more of the answers is correct. Choose

A. If 1, 2, and 3 are correct.
B. If only 1 and 3 are correct.
C. If only 2 and 4 are correct.
D. If only 4 is correct.
E. If all are correct.

14.11 Oral medications that are used to treat premature ejaculation include
1. Prostaglandin E_1.
2. Papaverine.
3. Phentolamine.
4. Clomipramine.

14.12 Among patients with a gender identity disorder, there is a high rate of comorbid
1. Borderline personality disorder.
2. Suicidal and self-destructive behavior.
3. Substance abuse disorders.
4. Bipolar disorder.

14.13 Psychotherapy for patients with gender identity disorder should
1. Help them see that they should not have surgical sex reassignment.
2. Be carried out on the basis of goals set by the patients.
3. Address concerns and fears about homosexuality that cause the disorder.
4. Help the patient adjust to the possibility of surgical sex reassignment.

14.14 A boy with thoughts of wanting to be a girl should be evaluated for
1. A gender identity disorder.
2. An adjustment disorder.
3. A mood disorder.
4. A psychotic disorder.

14.15 Which of the following are true about sexual function?
1. Dopamine enhances sexual function.
2. Serotonin enhances sexual function.
3. Serotonin decreases sexual function.
4. Dopamine decreases sexual function.

14.16 Which of the following may contribute to the development of sexual dysfunction?
1. Unconscious guilt and anxiety concerning sex.
2. History of sexual trauma.
3. Partners' failure to communicate to each other their sexual feelings and behaviors in which they want to engage.
4. Performance anxiety.

14.17 Hypoactive sexual desire
1. May be caused by anxiety about sexual activity.
2. May occur in one sexual context (e.g., with the individual's partner) but not another (e.g., self-directed masturbation).
3. Is relatively easy to treat.
4. May occur after the patient experiences difficulty with orgasm.

14.18 Treatments for premature ejaculation include
1. Intracavernous injection of papaverine and phentolamine.
2. The start-stop technique.
3. The squeeze technique.
4. Behavior therapy with negative reinforcement.

14.19 Vaginismus may be diagnosed with certainty only through
1. The clinical history from the patient.
2. Information from the patient's partner.
3. Lack of response to medication trials.
4. Gynecological examination.

14.20 Patients with paraphilias
1. Do not suffer significant distress due to the deviant sexual behavior.
2. Usually engage in only one type of deviant sexual behavior.
3. Usually develop the disorder before 18 years of age.
4. Are approximately 50% men and 50% women.

ANSWERS

14.1 The answer is **C**. Patients with borderline personality disorder have transient wishes to change gender because of their identity diffusion.

14.2 The answer is **C**. Gender identity is established by 3 years of age.

14.3 The answer is **E**. Medications that can interfere with sexual functioning include tricyclic antidepressants, monoamine oxidase inhibitors, selective serotonin reuptake inhibitors, and antipsychotic medications.

14.4 The answer is **E**. The incidence of gender identity disorder of childhood is unknown.

14.5 The answer is **E**. The treatment of gender identity disorder for a boy includes helping the boy avoid ostracism and humiliation, increasing the boy's comfort with his or her own sex, developing a close, trusting relationship between a male therapist and the boy, and stopping parental encouragement of feminine behaviors.

14.6 The answer is **D**. All of the following drugs or medications cause sexual dysfunction except bupropion (Wellbutrin).

14.7 The answer is **E**. The excitement stage in the sexual cycle is characterized by an increase in heart rate and blood pressure and erotic feelings that lead to vaginal lubrication in women and penile erection in men.

14.8 The answer is **D**. The prevalence of premature ejaculation for males in the general population is approximately 35%.

14.9 The answer is **C**. The primary treatment for a sexual aversion disorder is systematic desensitization, which helps reduce the patient's fear and avoidance.

14.10 The answer is **D**. The first step and most likely way for a woman with general anorgasmia to become orgasmic is a program of directed masturbation.

14.11 The answer is **D**. The oral medication that is used to treat premature ejaculation is clomipramine. The selective serotonin reuptake inhibitors also are being used.

14.12   The answer is **A.** Among patients with a gender identity disorder, there is a high rate of comorbid borderline personality disorder, suicidal and self-destructive behavior, and substance abuse disorders.

14.13   The answer is **C.** Psychotherapy for patients with gender identity disorder should be carried out on the basis of goals set by the patients and should help the patient adjust to the possibility of surgical sex reassignment.

14.14   The answer is **E.** A boy with thoughts of wanting to be a girl should be evaluated for gender identity disorder, an adjustment disorder, a mood disorder, and a psychotic disorder.

14.15   The answer is **B.** Dopamine enhances sexual function and serotonin decreases sexual function.

14.16   The answer is **E.** Sexual dysfunction may be caused by unconscious guilt and anxiety concerning sex, a history of sexual trauma, partners' failure to communicate to each other their sexual feelings and behaviors in which they want to engage, or performance anxiety.

14.17   The answer is **C.** Hypoactive sexual desire occurs in all sexual contexts (e.g., with a partner or alone). It rarely occurs after the patient experiences difficulty with orgasm. It may *not* be caused by anxiety about sexual activity (sexual aversion). It is the most difficult sexual disorder to treat.

14.18   The answer is **E.** A treatment for premature ejaculation includes intracavernous injection of papaverine and phentolamine, the start-stop technique, or the squeeze technique.

14.19   The answer is **D.** Vaginismus may be diagnosed with certainty only through gynecological examination.

14.20   The answer is **B.** Patients with paraphilias do not suffer significant distress due to the deviant sexual behavior and usually develop the disorder before 18 years of age. They usually engage in *many* types of deviant sexual behavior. Perpetrators are approximately 90% men and 10% women.

CHAPTER 15

ADJUSTMENT DISORDER

QUESTIONS

Directions: Select the single best response for each of the following questions:

15.1 One of the diagnostic criteria for adjustment disorders specifies onset of the symptoms within how many months of the stressor?
   A. 1 month.
   B. 2 months.
   C. 3 months.
   D. 6 months.
   E. 9 months.

15.2 Adjustment disorder with depressed mood or mixed mood is associated with which of the following findings compared with depressive disorders?
   A. Increased rate of suicide.
   B. Longer hospitalizations.
   C. Higher rate of relapse.
   D. More marital problems.
   E. More psychotic episodes.

15.3 A patient who, when diagnosed with cancer, denies the diagnosis of malignancy and does not comply with the recommended treatment may have
   A. Adjustment disorder not otherwise specified.
   B. Adjustment disorder with anxious mood.
   C. Adjustment disorder with physical complaints.
   D. Adjustment disorder with depressed mood.
   E. None of the above.

15.4 Which of the following is true?
   A. Adjustment disorder usually is the incipient phase of an emerging psychiatric disorder.

B. The long-term prognosis is better for adults than for adolescents with adjustment disorder.
C. Adults have fewer symptoms of depression with adjustment disorder than do adolescents.
D. All of the above.
E. None of the above.

15.5 The mean length of treatment for patients with adjustment disorder is
A. 2 months or less.
B. 3 months.
C. 4 months.
D. 5 months.
E. 6 months or more.

15.6 At 5-year follow-up, approximately what percentage of patients with adjustment disorder are completely well?
A. 10%.
B. 30%.
C. 50%.
D. 70%.
E. 90%.

Directions: For each of the statements below, one or more of the answers is correct. Choose

A. If 1, 2, and 3 are correct.
B. If only 1 and 3 are correct.
C. If only 2 and 4 are correct.
D. If only 4 is correct.
E. If all are correct.

15.7 Modifiers that have been shown to determine who will experience an adjustment disorder following stress include
1. Ego strength.
2. Social support system.
3. Underlying personality disorders.
4. Socioeconomic status.

15.8 Treatment of the adjustment disorder requires
1. Management of significant dysfunction created by the stressor.
2. Helping the patient avoid further stressors.

3. Prevention of deliberate self-harm.
4. Antidepressant medication.

15.9 Medication indicated for symptom reduction in patients with adjustment disorder includes
1. Mood stabilizers for mood swings.
2. Antipsychotics for relief of anxiety.
3. β-blockers for relief of anxiety.
4. Benzodiazepines for relief of anxiety and insomnia.

15.10 Psychosocial interventions for adjustment disorder include
1. Individual supportive psychotherapy.
2. Crises intervention counseling.
3. Group therapy.
4. Marital/couples therapy.

ANSWERS

15.1 The answer is **C.** One of the diagnostic criteria for adjustment disorders specifies onset of the symptoms within 3 months of the stressor.

15.2 The answer is **D.** Adjustment disorder with depressed mood or mixed mood is associated with more marital problems than depressive disorders.

15.3 The answer is **A.** A patient who, when diagnosed with cancer, denies the diagnosis of malignancy and does not comply with the recommended treatment may have adjustment disorder not otherwise specified.

15.4 The answer is **B.** The long-term prognosis is better for adults than for adolescents with adjustment disorder.

15.5 The answer is **E.** According to Despland et al. 1995,[*] the mean length of treatment for patients with adjustment disorders is more than 6 months.

15.6 The answer is **D.** At 5-year follow-up, approximately 70% of patients with adjustment disorder are completely well.

---

[*]Despland JN, Monod L, Ferrero F: Clinical relevance of adjustment disorder in DSM-III-R and DSM-IV. Compr Psychiatry 36:456–460, 1995.

15.7   The answer is **A.** Modifiers that have been shown to determine who will experience adjustment disorder following stress include ego strength, social support systems, and underlying personality disorders.

15.8   The answer is **A.** Treatment of the adjustment disorder requires management of significant dysfunction created by the stressor, helping the patient avoid further stressors, and prevention of deliberate self-harm. Antidepressant medication is not required and is rarely used.

15.9   The answer is **D.** Medication indicated for symptom reduction in patients with adjustment disorders includes benzodiazepines for relief of anxiety and insomnia. Mood stabilizers are not indicated for mood swings. Antipsychotics and β-blockers are not typically used for relief of anxiety in these patients.

15.10   The answer is **E.** Psychosocial interventions for adjustment disorder include individual supportive psychotherapy, crises intervention counseling, group therapy, and marital/couples therapy.

CHAPTER 16

IMPULSE CONTROL DISORDERS NOT ELSEWHERE CLASSIFIED

QUESTIONS

Directions: Select the single best response for each of the following questions:

16.1 The "dyscontrol syndrome" described by Mark and Ervin in 1970 included
   A. Physical assault.
   B. Pathological intoxication.
   C. Impulsive sexual behavior.
   D. Traffic violations and serious automobile accidents.
   E. All of the above.

16.2 Which of the following medications is approved by the Food and Drug Administration for treatment of aggressive behavior?
   A. Buspirone.
   B. β-blockers.
   C. Haloperidol.
   D. Valproic acid.
   E. None of the above.

16.3 The diagnostic criteria for kleptomania include
   A. Recurrent failure to resist impulses to steal objects that are needed for personal use.
   B. Increasing tension immediately after committing the theft.
   C. Pleasure or gratification at the time of committing the theft.
   D. Stealing committed to express anger.
   E. A and C.

16.4 Trichotillomania is most common among
   A. Preadolescent girls.
   B. Preadolescent boys.

       C. Female college students.
       D. Male college students.
       E. Adults.

16.5   Preliminary findings about the epidemiology of patients with kleptomania include all of the following **EXCEPT**
       A. A trend of the illness being more prevalent in females.
       B. The patient almost always has a psychosocial stressor.
       C. Mean duration of illness of approximately 15 years.
       D. Frequent comorbidity with depressive disorders.
       E. Frequent comorbidity with anxiety disorders.

16.6   The peak incidence of fire setting occurs at age
       A. 12.
       B. 17.
       C. 22.
       D. 27.
       E. 32.

16.7   The overall dropout rate for patients in treatment for pathological gambling at 1-year follow-up is approximately
       A. 20%.
       B. 40%.
       C. 60%.
       D. 80%.
       E. 100%.

16.8   Studies for the treatment of trichotillomania have shown a clear response to the medication
       A. Clomipramine.
       B. Fluoxetine.
       C. Sertraline.
       D. Paroxetine.
       E. Valproic acid.

Directions: For each of the statements below, one or more of the answers is correct. Choose

       A. If 1, 2, and 3 are correct.
       B. If only 1 and 3 are correct.
       C. If only 2 and 4 are correct.

D. If only 4 is correct.

E. If all are correct.

16.9   Which of the following is a clinical feature of pathological gambling?
1.   High risk taking.
2.   Inability to stop.
3.   Overconfidence.
4.   Chasing of losses.

16.10   Patients with episodic violent behavior often have a history of
1.   Head trauma.
2.   Attention-deficit/hyperactivity disorder.
3.   Substance abuse.
4.   Bipolar disorder.

16.11   Fire setting
1.   Occurs at a prevalence of approximately 35% in the general population.
2.   Comorbid with alcoholism is associated with a good prognosis.
3.   Is treated by biofeedback.
4.   As a symptom may be best understood as a communication from an individual with few social skills.

16.12   Pathological gambling and alcohol disorders have the following issues in common:
1.   Psychological symptoms in adjusting to abrupt discontinuation.
2.   Patients often overlook basic needs of sleep, food, and sex.
3.   Abstinence is a crucial part in recovery.
4.   Naltrexone reduces the frequency of undesirable behaviors.

16.13   Clues on physical examination that suggest a diagnosis of trichotillomania rather than a dermatologic disorder include
1.   Hair loss on the side of the body opposite to the dominant hand.
2.   Within the area of hair loss, broken hairs are of basically equal length.
3.   No changes occur in the nails except perhaps for signs of biting.
4.   Failure of the hair to grow back even once the behavior has been curtailed.

16.14   Which of the following impulse control disorders occurs more commonly in females then males?
1.   Pathological gambling.
2.   Trichotillomania.
3.   Pyromania.
4.   Kleptomania.

16.15   Trichotillomania also may be a symptom of
  1.   Major depressive disorder.
  2.   Obsessive-compulsive disorder.
  3.   Borderline personality disorder.
  4.   Mental retardation.

ANSWERS

16.1   The answer is **E**. The "dyscontrol syndrome" described by Mark and Ervin in 1970 included physical assault, impulsive sexual behavior, traffic violations and serious automobile accidents, and pathological intoxication.

16.2   The answer is **E**. No medication has been approved by the Food and Drug Administration for treatment of aggressive behavior.

16.3   The answer is **C**. The diagnostic criteria for kleptomania include pleasure or gratification at the time of committing the theft. Also included in the criteria are recurrent failures to resist impulses to steal objects that are not needed for personal use, increasing tension immediately *before* committing the theft, and stealing committed is *not* done to express anger.

16.4   The answer is **A**. Trichotillomania is most common among preadolescent girls.

16.5   The answer is **B**. Preliminary findings about the epidemiology of patients with kleptomania show the patient rarely has a psychosocial stressor, which is different than those who shoplift and do not have a diagnosis of kleptomania.

16.6   The answer is **B**. The peak incidence of fire setting occurs at age 17.

16.7   The answer is **D**. The overall dropout rate for patients in treatment for pathological gambling at 1-year follow-up is approximately 80%.

16.8   The answer is **A**. Studies for the treatment of trichotillomania have shown a clear response to the medication clomipramine.

16.9   The answer is **E**. Clinical features of pathological gambling are high risk taking, inability to stop, overconfidence, and chasing of losses.

16.10   The answer is **A**. Patients with episodic violent behavior often have a history of head trauma, attention-deficit/hyperactivity disorder, and substance abuse.

16.11   The answer is **D.** Fire setting as a symptom may be best understood as a communication from an individual with few social skills. Its prevalence in the general population is unknown. Fire setting comorbid with alcoholism (or mental retardation) is associated with a poor prognosis.

16.12   The answer is **A.** Pathological gambling and alcohol disorders have the following issues in common: psychological symptoms in adjusting to abrupt discontinuation; patients often overlook basic needs of sleep, food, and sex; and abstinence is a crucial part in recovery. Naltrexone reduces the frequency of craving for alcohol and the number of drinking days, but has not been assessed for efficacy in pathological gambling.

16.13   The answer is **B.** Clues on physical examination that suggest a diagnosis of trichotillomania rather than a dermatologic disorder include hair loss on the side of the body opposite to the dominant hand and no changes in the nails except perhaps for signs of biting. Within the area of hair loss, broken hairs are of *unequal* length. The hair typically grows back once the behavior has been curtailed.

16.14   The answer is **B.** Trichotillomania and kleptomania appear to occur more commonly in females than males. Pathological gambling and pyromania occur more frequently in men.

16.15   The answer is **E.** Trichotillomania also may be a symptom of major depressive disorder, obsessive-compulsive disorder, borderline personality disorder, or mental retardation.

CHAPTER 17
PERSONALITY DISORDERS

Directions: Select the single best response for each of the following questions:

17.1 The percentage of mental health outpatients with a personality disorder is
   A. Less than 10%–15%.
   B. 10%–20%.
   C. 20%–29%.
   D. 30%–50%.
   E. More than 50%.

17.2 Patients with schizoid personality disorder may benefit from
   A. Supportive therapy.
   B. Insight-oriented therapy.
   C. Cognitive therapy.
   D. Group therapy.
   E. All of the above.

17.3 Which of the following is not a symptom of both schizotypal personality disorder and schizophrenia?
   A. A persistent pattern of social and interpersonal deficits.
   B. Ideas of reference.
   C. Magical thinking.
   D. Fixed false beliefs (i.e., delusions).
   E. Paranoid ideation.

17.4 All of the following are diagnostic criteria for paranoid personality disorder **EXCEPT**
   A. Reluctance to confide in others.
   B. Persistently bears grudges.
   C. Reading hidden threatening meanings into benign remarks.

    D. Almost always choosing solitary activities.

    E. Preoccupation with unjustified doubts about friends' loyalty.

17.5   The most prevalent Axis II disorder is

    A. Paranoid personality disorder.

    B. Narcissistic personality disorder.

    C. Borderline personality disorder.

    D. Antisocial personality disorder.

    E. Histrionic personality disorder.

17.6   Which of the following is **FALSE** regarding borderline personality disorder?

    A. It results from a failure to resolve the oedipal conflict between ages 3 and 5.

    B. Its prevalence is 2%–3% of the population.

    C. Its central characteristic is impaired capacity for attachment.

    D. Patients suffer from intense rage and self-hatred.

    E. Long-term therapy is indicated for treatment.

17.7   Avoidant personality disorder develops from

    A. Parental neglect of their fears, failures, or dependency.

    B. Parental mismanagement of the 2- to 3-year-old child's efforts to become autonomous.

    C. Parental overindulgence of the child.

    D. Parental rejection and censure of the child, which may be reinforced by rejecting peers.

    E. All of the above.

17.8   Obsessive-compulsive personality disorder develops from

    A. Parental attempts to socialize the child (e.g., toilet training).

    B. Parental neglect of their fears, failures, or dependency.

    C. Parental mismanagement of the 2- to 3-year-old child's efforts to become autonomous.

    D. Parental overindulgence of the child.

    E. None of the above.

Directions: For each of the statements below, one or more of the answers is correct. Choose

    A. If 1, 2, and 3 are correct.

    B. If only 1 and 3 are correct.

    C. If only 2 and 4 are correct.

    D. If only 4 is correct.

    E. If all are correct.

17.9 Diagnosis of a personality disorder is best made
   1. By interviewing the patient 1–2 times.
   2. By using collateral information.
   3. By interviewing the patient in the midst of a depressive episode.
   4. By using a semi-structured or structured instrument.

17.10 Which of the following personality disorders responds to pharmacologic treatment?
   1. Narcissistic personality disorder.
   2. Schizotypal personality disorder.
   3. Histrionic personality disorder.
   4. Borderline personality disorder.

17.11 Which of the following treatments are appropriate for patients with avoidant personality disorder?
   1. Assertiveness training.
   2. Cognitive therapy that challenges pathological assumptions.
   3. Selective serotonin reuptake inhibitors (SSRIs).
   4. Antipsychotic medication.

ANSWERS

17.1 The answer is **D**. The percentage of outpatients with a personality disorder is 30%–50%.

17.2 The answer is **E**. Patients with schizoid personality disorder may benefit from supportive, insight-oriented, cognitive, and group therapy.

17.3 The answer is **D**. Schizotypal patients do *not* have fixed false beliefs (i.e., delusions). Patients with schizotypal personality disorder and schizophrenia may have a persistent pattern of social and interpersonal deficits, ideas of reference, magical thinking, and paranoid ideation.

17.4 The answer is **D**. Diagnostic criteria for paranoid personality disorder do not include choosing solitary activities. The criteria include reluctance to confide in others, persistently bearing grudges, reading hidden threatening meanings into benign remarks, and preoccupation with unjustified doubts about friends' loyalty.

17.5 The answer is **C**. The most prevalent Axis II disorder is borderline personality disorder.

17.6   The answer is **A.** Borderline personality disorder does not result from a failure to resolve the oedipal conflict between ages 3 and 5. It is believed to result from mismanagement of the 2- to 3-year-old child's efforts to become autonomous.

17.7   The answer is **D.** Avoidant personality disorder develops from parental rejection and censure, which may be reinforced by rejecting peers.

17.8   The answer is **A.** Obsessive-compulsive personality disorder develops from parental attempts to socialize the child (e.g., toilet training).

17.9   The answer is **C.** Diagnosis of a personality disorder is best made by using collateral information, interviewing the patient several times, using a semi-structured or structured interview, and assessing the patient when *not* in the midst of an acute mood episode.

17.10   The answer is **C.** Schizotypal personality disorder and borderline personality disorder respond to pharmacological treatment.

17.11   The answer is **A.** Assertiveness training and SSRIs are appropriate for patients with avoidant personality disorder. Antipsychotic medication is not indicated.

CHAPTER 18

DISORDERS USUALLY FIRST DIAGNOSED IN INFANCY, CHILDHOOD, OR ADOLESCENCE

Directions: Select the single best response for each of the following questions:

18.1   The most common diagnosis of child and adolescent patients is
    A.   Conduct disorder.
    B.   Attention-deficit/hyperactivity disorder (ADHD).
    C.   Separation anxiety disorder.
    D.   Stuttering.
    E.   Mathematics disorder.

18.2   Symptoms of inattention common to ADHD include
    A.   Not appearing to listen when spoken to directly.
    B.   Not following through on instructions, chores, or homework.
    C.   Difficulty organizing tasks.
    D.   Losing things.
    E.   All of the above.

18.3   Which of the following disorders is comorbid in 25% of ADHD patients?
    A.   Tourette's disorder.
    B.   Bipolar disorder.
    C.   Conduct disorder.
    D.   A and C.
    E.   All of the above.

18.4   Which is true about the course and prognosis of ADHD?
    A.   Inattention lessens during childhood and adolescence.
    B.   ADHD is a basically benign and self-limited childhood disorder.

C. Follow-up studies reveal that 50% of children with ADHD eventually develop antisocial personality disorder.
D. The prevalence of ADHD is estimated to decline by 50% about every 5 years until the mid-20s.
E. All of the above.

18.5   Environmental management of ADHD includes
A. Encouraging several friends to visit the home.
B. Discouraging fine motor exercises like puzzles.
C. Keeping toys dispersed in the room instead of the closet.
D. Decorating with bright colors.
E. None of the above.

18.6   Which of the following statements is true regarding ADHD?
A. Attention effects of psychostimulants appear to be dose dependent.
B. Behavioral effects of psychostimulants appear to be dose dependent.
C. Many patients show tolerance to the effects of psychostimulants.
D. Nonstimulant medications treat inattention as well as psychostimulants.
E. All of the above.

18.7   Minors (younger than 18 years) are responsible for what percentage of violent crimes?
A. 5%.
B. 10%.
C. 20%.
D. 30%.
E. 40%.

18.8   The most common genetically based cause of moderate and severe mental retardation is
A. Trisomy 21 (Down's syndrome).
B. Fragile X syndrome.
C. Phenylketonuria.
D. Tuberous sclerosis.
E. None of the above.

18.9   Learning disorders are defined to exclude individuals whose slow learning is explainable by
A. Motor or sensory handicaps.
B. Weak educational opportunities.
C. Low intelligence.

    D. All of the above.

    E. None of the above.

18.10 A patient with Tourette's disorder may have

    A. Motor but not vocal tics.

    B. Vocal but not motor tics.

    C. Both motor and vocal tics.

    D. Dyskinesias.

    E. Dystonias.

18.11 The most common type of learning disorder is

    A. Reading disorder.

    B. Writing disorder.

    C. Arithmetic disorder.

    D. Spelling disorder.

    E. All types are approximately equal in frequency.

18.12 Mild mental retardation is characterized by

    A. An IQ between 45–55.

    B. A life span of approximately 20 years.

    C. A second grade academic level.

    D. Ability to manage a job.

    E. All of the above.

18.13 A good prognostic indicator for a child with autism is

    A. Later onset.

    B. High IQ.

    C. Good vocabulary.

    D. A and C.

    E. All of the above.

18.14 Tics are

    A. Typically seen during periods of increased stress or excitement.

    B. A common symptom of depression.

    C. Responsive to cognitive therapy.

    D. Not exacerbated by psychostimulants.

    E. All of the above.

18.15 Treatments effective for encopresis include

    A. Laxatives.

    B. Counseling.

C. Anal sphincter feedback.
D. All of the above.
E. None of the above.

Directions: For each of the statements below, one or more of the answers is correct. Choose

A. If 1, 2, and 3 are correct.
B. If only 1 and 3 are correct.
C. If only 2 and 4 are correct.
D. If only 4 is correct.
E. If all are correct.

18.16 Psychostimulant treatment of children with ADHD generally leads to which of the following outcomes?
1. Reduced inattention.
2. Improved academic performance.
3. Reduced impulsivity.
4. Decreased criminal behavior.

18.17 Which of the following behaviors is characteristic of a child with oppositional defiant disorder
1. Intimidates or bullies others.
2. Often loses temper.
3. Initiates physical fights.
4. Deliberately annoys people.

18.18 Symptoms of hyperactivity and impulsivity from ADHD include
1. Blurting out answers before questions have been asked.
2. Fidgeting.
3. Running about and climbing excessively.
4. Fire setting with intention to cause damage.

18.19 In contrast with children with the hyperactivity type of ADHD, those with the inattention type
1. Have more anxiety and shyness.
2. Have less comorbid depression.
3. Have less comorbid conduct disorder.
4. Have a better response to clonidine than psychostimulants.

18.20 Common medical causes of ADHD-like symptoms include
1. Streptococcal infection.
2. Hyperthyroidism.
3. Constipation.
4. Theophylline.

18.21 A norepinephrine hypothesis of ADHD is supported by
1. High levels of 3-methoxy-4-hydroxyphenylglycol (MHPG).
2. Therapeutic effects of tricyclic antidepressants and monoamine oxidase inhibitors.
3. A low spontaneous blink rate.
4. Effectiveness of the α_2 agonists clonidine and guanfacine.

18.22 The differential diagnosis for a child with fidgeting and talking excessively includes
1. Physical or sexual trauma.
2. Depression.
3. ADHD.
4. Bipolar disorder.

18.23 Common features of conduct disorder include
1. Cruelty to animals.
2. Impulsivity.
3. Shoplifting.
4. Stealing from the rich to give to the poor.

18.24 The natural course of conduct disorder is improved by
1. Marriage to a stable spouse.
2. Lengthy incarceration.
3. Support from family and friends.
4. Religious involvement.

18.25 The etiology of oppositional defiant disorder is related to
1. Parental problems.
2. Identification by the child with an impulse-disordered parent.
3. Attachment deficits caused by parents' emotional or physical unavailability.
4. Deficits in dopamine transmission.

18.26 Reading disordered children typically have problems with
1. Left-right orientation.
2. Letter reversals.

    3. Substitution (e.g., truck, trick).
    4. Spelling.

18.27 Reading disorder is improved by
    1. Methods of improving the child's self-esteem.
    2. Vitamin and dietary approaches.
    3. Parental involvement in the educational program.
    4. Psychostimulants.

18.28 Stuttering improves
    1. Spontaneously in 50%–80% of cases.
    2. With intensive electromyography feedback.
    3. With modification of environmental triggers.
    4. With home-based smooth speech therapy.

18.29 For patients with mental retardation, behavior modification can be used to treat
    1. Aggressive behavior.
    2. Self-injury.
    3. Asocial behavior.
    4. Low self-esteem.

18.30 Treatment for autistic disorder includes
    1. Counseling for parents.
    2. Long-term supervision and structure.
    3. Antipsychotic medication for disruptive behavior.
    4. Anticonvulsants or psychostimulants for disruptive behavior.

ANSWERS

18.1   The answer is **A.** The most common diagnosis of child and adolescent patients is conduct disorder.

18.2   The answer is **E.** Symptoms of inattention common to ADHD include not appearing to listen when spoken to directly and not following through on instructions, chores, or homework. Children also have difficulty organizing tasks and commonly lose things.

18.3   The answer is **E.** Tourette's disorder, bipolar disorder, and conduct disorder are comorbid in 25% of ADHD patients.

18.4   The answer is **D**. The prevalence of ADHD is estimated to decline by 50% about every 5 years until the mid-20s. Hyperactivity and impulsivity (not inattention) lessen during childhood and adolescence. Follow-up studies reveal that 25% of children with ADHD eventually develop antisocial personality disorder.

18.5   The answer is **E**. Environmental management of ADHD includes encouraging *one* friend to visit the home, *encouraging* fine motor exercises like puzzles, keeping toys in the closet, and decorating with *subdued* colors.

18.6   The answer is **B**. Behavioral effects of psychostimulants appear to be dose-dependent, but attention effects of psychostimulants are not. Only a small percentage of patients became tolerant to the effects of psychostimulants. Nonstimulant medications do not treat inattention as well as psychostimulants.

18.7   The answer is **C**. Minors (younger than 18 years) are responsible for 20% of violent crimes.

18.8   The answer is **A**. The most common genetically based cause of moderate and severe mental retardation is trisomy 21.

18.9   The answer is **D**. Learning disorders are defined to *exclude* individuals whose slow learning is explainable by motor or sensory handicaps, weak educational opportunities, and low intelligence.

18.10   The answer is **C**. A patient with Tourette's disorder may have both motor and vocal tics.

18.11   The answer is **A**. The most common type of learning disorder is reading disorder.

18.12   The answer is **D**. Mild mental retardation is characterized by ability to manage a job. Patients have an IQ between 55–70 and a sixth grade academic level with a life span of approximately 50 years.

18.13   The answer is **E**. Good prognostic indicators for a child with autism are later onset, high IQ, and good vocabulary.

18.14   The answer is **A**. Tics are typically seen during periods of increased stress or excitement. Tics may be exacerbated by psychostimulants.

18.15   The answer is **D**. Treatments effective for encopresis include laxatives, counseling, and anal sphincter feedback.

18.16   The answer is **B**. Psychostimulant treatment of children with ADHD generally leads to reduced inattention and reduced impulsivity, but not improved academic performance (as formally measured) or decreased criminal behavior.

18.17   The answer is **C**. A child with oppositional defiant disorder typically often loses his or her temper and deliberately annoys people.

18.18   The answer is **A**. Symptoms of hyperactivity and impulsivity from ADHD include blurting out answers before questions have been asked, fidgeting, and running about and climbing excessively. Conduct disorder patients may be involved with fire setting with intention to cause damage.

18.19   The answer is **B**. In contrast with children with the hyperactivity type of ADHD, those with the inattention type have more anxiety and shyness and they have less comorbid conduct disorder. They have *more* comorbid depression and are *less* responsive to clonidine than psychostimulants.

18.20   The answer is **E**. Common medical causes of ADHD-like symptoms include streptococcal infection, hyperthyroidism, constipation, and theophylline.

18.21   The answer is **C**. A norepinephrine hypothesis of ADHD is supported by therapeutic effects of tricyclic antidepressants, monoamine oxidase inhibitors, and the α_2 agonists clonidine and guanfacine. Low levels of MHPG support the hypothesis. A low spontaneous blink rate, which correlates with dopamine function rather than norepinephrine function, is noted in some schizophrenic patients.

18.22   The answer is **E**. The differential diagnosis for a child who fidgets and talks excessively includes physical or sexual trauma, depression, ADHD, and bipolar disorder.

18.23   The answer is **B**. Common features of conduct disorder include cruelty to animals and shoplifting. Impulsivity is notably absent in conduct disorder, and these patients do not steal to help others, per se.

18.24   The answer is **B**. The natural course of conduct disorder is improved by marriage to a stable spouse and support from family and friends. Lengthy incarceration and religious involvement do not appear to improve the course.

18.25   The answer is **A**. The etiology of oppositional defiant disorder is related to parental problems, identification by the child with an impulse-disordered parent, and attachment deficits caused by parents' emotional or physical unavailability. Abnormalities in dopaminergic transmission have not been noted.

18.26   The answer is **E**. Reading disordered children typically have problems with left-right orientation, letter reversals, substitution (e.g., truck, trick), and spelling.

18.27   The answer is **B**. Reading disorder is improved by methods of improving the child's self-esteem and parental involvement in the educational program. Vitamin, dietary, and psychotropic medication approaches have not been shown to be helpful.

18.28   The answer is **E**. Stuttering improves spontaneously in 50%–80% of cases. Stuttering responds to therapies of intensive electromyography feedback, modification of environmental triggers, and home-based smooth speech therapy.

18.29   The answer is **A**. For patients with mental retardation, behavior modification can be used to treat aggressive behavior, self-injury, and asocial behavior.

18.30   The answer is **E**. Treatment for autistic disorder includes counseling for parents, long-term supervision and structure, and antipsychotic, anticonvulsant or psychostimulant medication for disruptive behavior.

CHAPTER 19

SLEEP DISORDERS

QUESTIONS

Directions: Select the single best response for each of the following questions:

19.1 All of the following are dyssomnias **EXCEPT**
A. Narcolepsy.
B. Sleepwalking disorder.
C. Primary hypersomnia.
D. Circadian rhythm sleep disorder.
E. Primary insomnia.

19.2 Sleep disorders have been found to be associated with
A. Poor job performance.
B. Accidents.
C. Impaired physical well-being.
D. Increased use of alcohol.
E. All of the above.

19.3 Treatments for chronic insomnia include all of the following **EXCEPT**
A. Relaxation therapies.
B. Biofeedback.
C. Sleep deprivation therapy.
D. Behavior modification regarding cues associated with arousal.
E. Sleep restriction therapy.

19.4 Circadian rhythm sleep disorders
A. Are not associated with significant medical comorbidity.
B. Are not associated with impairment in psychosocial functioning.
C. Are commonly comorbid with schizophrenia.
D. Appear to cause more cognitive errors in physicians and air traffic controllers who work at night.
E. Are not associated with increased rates of injury for rotating shift workers.

19.5   Which medication used to treat insomnia that is least prone to cause confusion in elderly patients?
   A.   Tricyclic antidepressants.
   B.   Trazodone.
   C.   Diphenhydramine.
   D.   Zolpidem.
   E.   Thioridazine.

19.6   Treatment for sleepwalking disorder and sleep terror disorder usually involves
   A.   Reducing stress and anxiety.
   B.   Sleep deprivation.
   C.   Behavior therapy.
   D.   Benzodiazepines.
   E.   All of the above.

19.7   Sleep disturbance in patients with general anxiety disorder
   A.   Is similar to that experienced with depression.
   B.   Involves increased REM latency.
   C.   Involves increased sleep latency.
   D.   Involves both increased REM and sleep latency.
   E.   All of the above.

19.8   Acute alcohol administration causes
   A.   Increased sleep latency.
   B.   Decreased REM sleep and arousals in the first half of the night.
   C.   Increased REM sleep and arousals in the second half of the night.
   D.   Increased sleep efficiency.
   E.   None of the above.

Directions: For each of the statements below, one or more of the answers is correct. Choose

   A.   If 1, 2, and 3 are correct.
   B.   If only 1 and 3 are correct.
   C.   If only 2 and 4 are correct.
   D.   If only 4 is correct.
   E.   If all are correct.

19.9   The sleep of elderly patients is characterized by
   1.   Fewer sleep stage shifts.
   2.   Lighter depth.

3. More slow-wave sleep.
4. More transient arousals.

19.10 Apnea is associated with which of the following?
1. Loud snoring.
2. Cardiac arrhythmias.
3. Obesity.
4. Schizophrenia.

19.11 Which of the following statements are true about sleep?
1. During wakefulness, the EEG is characterized by low-voltage activity consisting of a mix of alpha and beta frequencies.
2. The beta rhythm disappears in Stage 1.
3. Stage 2 consists of sleep spindles and K complexes.
4. Stages 3 and 4 have high-amplitude alpha bands.

19.12 Which of the following statements are true regarding the changes in sleep during the life cycle?
1. No changes occur in sleep efficiency throughout the life cycle.
2. Sleep in prepubertal children is characterized by large percentages of REM.
3. Contrary to popular belief, with advancing age, naps are not more frequent.
4. Slow wave is decreased in adolescence in relation to a rapid period of synaptic pruning (apoptosis).

19.13 A thorough history regarding sleep problems includes
1. The patient's description of what constitutes healthy sleep.
2. A two-week sleep log.
3. A log regarding the use of stimulants, hypnotics, and alcohol.
4. A log regarding consumption of carbohydrates.

19.14 Practice guidelines for the use of stimulants in narcolepsy dictate that
1. Diagnosis of narcolepsy should be established by polysomnogram and the Multiple Sleep Latency Test.
2. Modafinil has proven efficacy for narcolepsy.
3. The maximum methylphenidate dose should be 100 mg.
4. Medications approved for narcolepsy are safe during pregnancy and breast feeding.

19.15   Which of the following are true about sleep and mood disorders?
1.   Patients with insomnia have a higher risk of developing depression at follow-up.
2.   Patients with depression have sleep fragmentation and increased REM in the first half of the night.
3.   Patients with mania have abnormalities that are very similar to those with depression.
4.   Patients with depression have changes in sleep that persist after resolution of the episode.

ANSWERS

19.1   The answer is **B.** Dyssomnias include narcolepsy, primary hypersomnia, circadian rhythm sleep disorder, and primary insomnia. Sleepwalking disorder is a parasomnia.

19.2   The answer is **E.** Sleep disorders have been found to be associated with poor job performance, accidents, impaired physical well-being, and increased use of alcohol.

19.3   The answer is **C.** Treatments for chronic insomnia do not include sleep deprivation therapy but do include relaxation therapies, biofeedback, behavior modification regarding cues associated with arousal, and sleep restriction therapy.

19.4   The answer is **D.** Circadian rhythm sleep disorders appear to cause more cognitive errors in physicians and air traffic controllers who work at night. The disorders are associated with significant medical comorbidity, impairment in psychosocial functioning, and increased rates of injury for rotating shift workers.

19.5   The answer is **B.** The medication used to treat insomnia that is least prone to cause confusion in elderly patients is trazodone. Zolpidem, benzodiazepines, and medications with significant anticholinergic action (tricyclic antidepressants, diphenhydramine, and thioridazine) often cause confusion.

19.6   The answer is **A.** Treatment for sleepwalking disorder and sleep terror disorder usually involves reducing stress and anxiety, which exacerbate these disorders.

19.7   The answer is **C.** Sleep disturbance in patients with general anxiety disorder involves increased sleep latency.

19.8   The answer is **C.** Acute alcohol administration causes increased REM sleep and arousals in the second half of the night. It also causes *decreased* sleep latency and efficiency.

19.9   The answer is **C.** The sleep of elderly patients is characterized by lighter depth and more transient arousals.

19.10   The answer is **A.** Apnea is associated with loud snoring, cardiac arrhythmias, and obesity.

19.11   The answer is **B.** During wakefulness, the EEG is characterized by low-voltage activity consisting of a mix of alpha and beta frequencies. The *alpha* rhythm disappears in Stage 1. Stage 2 consists of sleep spindles and K complexes. Stages 3 and 4 have high-amplitude *delta* bands.

19.12   The answer is **C.** Sleep in prepubertal children is characterized by large percentages of REM. Slow wave is decreased in adolescence in relation to a rapid period of synaptic pruning. With advancing age, naps are indeed more frequent. In addition, sleep efficiency generally decreases over the life cycle.

19.13   The answer is **A.** A thorough history regarding sleep problems includes the patient's description of what constitutes healthy sleep, a two-week sleep log, and use of stimulants, hypnotics, and alcohol.

19.14   The answer is **A.** Practice guidelines for the use of stimulants in narcolepsy include that the diagnosis of narcolepsy should be established by polysomnogram and the Multiple Sleep Latency Test, modafinil has proven efficacy for narcolepsy, and the maximum methylphenidate dose should be 100 mg. It is not clear if medications approved for narcolepsy are safe during pregnancy and breast-feeding.

19.15   The answer is **E.** All of the following are true about sleep and mood disorders: patients with insomnia have a higher risk of developing depression at follow-up; patients with depression have sleep fragmentation and increased REM in the first half of the night; patients with depression have changes in sleep that persist after resolution of the episode; and patients with mania have abnormalities that are very similar to those with depression.

CHAPTER 20

EATING DISORDERS: ANOREXIA NERVOSA, BULIMIA NERVOSA, AND OBESITY

QUESTIONS

Directions: Select the single best response for each of the following questions:

20.1 Medical complications of anorexia nervosa include all of the following **EXCEPT**
- A. Leukopenia.
- B. Hypokalemic acidosis.
- C. Arrhythmia.
- D. Decreased renal function.
- E. Fatty degeneration of the liver.

20.2 Stress-induced eating is probably driven by activation of
- A. The opioid system.
- B. Thyrotropin-releasing hormone.
- C. Gastrin-releasing peptide.
- D. β_2-adrenergic receptors.
- E. α_2-adrenergic receptors.

20.3 All of the following stimulate feeding **EXCEPT**
- A. Corticotropin-releasing factor.
- B. Norepinephrine.
- C. Neuropeptide Y.
- D. α_2 agonists.
- E. All of the above.

20.4   The mortality rate at 10 years for patients with anorexia nervosa is approximately
      A. 2%.
      B. 7%.
      C. 12%.
      D. 17%.
      E. 22%.

20.5   The majority of bulimic patients
      A. Have obsessive-compulsive symptoms.
      B. Have signs and symptoms of depression.
      C. Have a history of anorexia.
      D. Have Russell's sign.
      E. All of the above.

20.6   The prevalence of bulimia nervosa in the general population is approximately
      A. 0.5%.
      B. 2%.
      C. 5%.
      D. 10%.
      E. 15%.

20.7   In patients with bulimia nervosa, antidepressant medication
      A. Is the treatment of choice.
      B. Is better than cognitive-behavioral therapy.
      C. Reduces binge-eating episodes.
      D. Has been proven effective in long-term studies.
      E. All of the above.

Directions: For each of the statements below, one or more of the answers is correct. Choose

      A. If 1, 2, and 3 are correct.
      B. If only 1 and 3 are correct.
      C. If only 2 and 4 are correct.
      D. If only 4 is correct.
      E. If all are correct.

20.8   The most effective treatment for mild obesity includes
      1. Exercise.
      2. Psychotherapy.

      3.   A balanced diet.

      4.   A medically supervised protein-sparing modified fast.

20.9   Physiological variables that affect eating include

      1.   Neuropeptide levels.

      2.   Metabolic rate.

      3.   Sensory receptors for taste and smell.

      4.   Condition of the gastrointestinal tract.

20.10   Anorectic patients often

      1.   Collect recipes.

      2.   Hoard large quantities of candies.

      3.   Prepare elaborate meals for their families.

      4.   Express intense fear about the onset of amenorrhea.

20.11   Which of the following treatments is indicated for a 17-year-old female with anorexia nervosa?

      1.   Behavior therapy to gain weight.

      2.   Family therapy.

      3.   Cognitive therapy to evaluate automatic thoughts.

      4.   Group therapy.

20.12   Binge-eating in bulimic patients

      1.   Often follows a period of dieting.

      2.   Is often accompanied by impulsive stealing.

      3.   Is usually followed by self-induced vomiting.

      4.   Usually occurs 1–2 times per month.

20.13   During a psychiatric interview, you discover a female patient had a binge-eating episode. On further evaluation, she could have

      1.   Binge-eating disorder.

      2.   Anorexia nervosa.

      3.   Bulimia nervosa.

      4.   No disorder.

20.14   Complications of obesity may include

      1.   Hypertension.

      2.   Congestive heart failure.

      3.   Diabetes mellitus.

      4.   Pulmonary dysfunction.

20.15 Standard treatment for obesity includes
   1. Behavior modification.
   2. Fenfluramine.
   3. Exercise.
   4. Antidepressant medication.

ANSWERS

20.1   The answer is **D.** Decreased renal function is not typically a medical complication of anorexia nervosa.

20.2   The answer is **A.** Stress-induced eating is probably driven by activation of the opioid system.

20.3   The answer is **A.** Corticotropin-releasing factor *inhibits* feeding.

20.4   The answer is **B.** The mortality rate at 10 years for patients with anorexia nervosa is approximately 7%.

20.5   The answer is **B.** The majority of bulimic patients have signs and symptoms of depression.

20.6   The answer is **B.** The prevalence of bulimia nervosa in the general population is approximately 2%.

20.7   The answer is **C.** Antidepressant medication reduces binge-eating episodes. Cognitive-behavioral therapy is the treatment of choice. The efficacy of antidepressant medication has not been studied with regard to bulimia nervosa.

20.8   The answer is **B.** The most effective treatment for mild obesity includes exercise and a balanced diet.

20.9   The answer is **E.** Physiological variables that affect eating include neuropeptide levels, metabolic rate, sensory receptors for taste and smell, and condition of the gastrointestinal tract.

20.10 The answer is **A.** Anorectic patients often collect recipes, hoard large amounts of candies, and prepare elaborate meals for their families. They do not express intense fear about the onset of amenorrhea.

20.11   The answer is **A.** A 17-year-old female with anorexia nervosa should receive behavior therapy to gain weight, cognitive therapy to evaluate automatic
thoughts, and family therapy. Group therapy has not proven useful for
anorectic patients, as it has for bulimia nervosa patients.

20.12   The answer is **A.** Binge-eating in bulimic patients often follows a period of diet-
ing, is often accompanied by impulsive stealing, and is usually followed by
self-induced vomiting. By definition it occurs at least twice per week for
3 months.

20.13   The answer is **E.** During a psychiatric interview, you discover a patient had a
binge-eating episode. On further evaluation, she could have binge-eating disorder, anorexia nervosa, bulimia nervosa, or no psychiatric disorder.

20.14   The answer is **E.** Complications of obesity may include hypertension, conges-
tive heart failure, diabetes mellitus, and (in severe obesity) pulmonary dysfunction.

20.15   The answer is **B.** Standard treatment for obesity includes behavior modification and exercise. Antidepressant medication is not indicated, and fenfluramine
was taken off the market because of potential cardiac side effects.

CHAPTER 21

PAIN DISORDERS

QUESTIONS

Directions: Select the single best response for each of the following questions:

21.1   Which disorders are more common in the first-degree relatives of patients with chronic pain?
A. Depression.
B. Anorexia.
C. Alcohol dependence.
D. Alzheimer's disease.
E. A and C.

21.2   According to the gate control theory, transmission of nerve impulses from the periphery to the spinal cord is modified by a gate-like mechanism located in the
A. Substantia gelatinosa.
B. Dorsal horn.
C. A-beta fibers.
D. A-delta fibers.
E. C fibers.

21.3   A simple measure of pain is provided by
A. The Minnesota Multiphasic Personality Inventory's hypochondriasis scale.
B. The McGill Pain Questionnaire.
C. The West Haven-Yale Multidimensional Pain Inventory.
D. The visual analog scale.
E. None of the above.

21.4   Which of the following statements about pain is **FALSE?**
A. Pain is a subjective problem and patient self-report is the mainstay of collecting the history.

B. Some patients in the intensive care unit, who have mental status changes, generally are unable to report pain.
C. Elderly patients generally feel less pain than adult patients.
D. Elderly patients are more susceptible to side effects of pain medication than adult patients.
E. Nonverbal scales are useful to assess pain.

21.5 In a patient without a history of alcohol or substance disorder, the risk of developing an addiction to pain medicine is
A. Zero.
B. Minimal.
C. Medium.
D. High.
E. Very high.

21.6 The goal of operant conditioning as a treatment for chronic pain is to
A. Reduce the patient's false assumptions about pain.
B. Allow the patient to opt out of situations that may worsen the pain.
C. Reinforce positive or "healthy" behaviors and to diminish destructive behaviors.
D. Facilitate use of medication for pain complaints.
E. None of the above.

21.7 According to controlled studies, which of the following treatments has been found effective in reducing **CHRONIC** pain?
A. Relaxation therapy.
B. Imagery.
C. Hypnosis.
D. A and C.
E. All of the above.

21.8 Which of the following is most efficacious in the treatment of pain related to neuropathies?
A. Neuroleptics.
B. Anticonvulsants.
C. Lithium.
D. Tricyclic antidepressants.
E. Benzodiazepines.

21.9 For mild or moderate postoperative pain, the medication of choice is
A. A nonsteroidal anti-inflammatory drug (NSAID) or acetaminophen.
B. An opioid analgesic.

    C. A tricyclic antidepressant.
    D. A selective serotonin reuptake inhibitor (SSRI).
    E. All of the above.

21.10 SSRIs reduce the efficacy of which pain medication by inhibiting its metabolism to an active medication in the liver?
    A. Naproxen.
    B. Acetaminophen.
    C. Codeine.
    D. Morphine sulfate.
    E. Meperidine.

Directions: For each of the statements below, one or more of the answers is correct. Choose

    A. If 1, 2, and 3 are correct.
    B. If only 1 and 3 are correct.
    C. If only 2 and 4 are correct.
    D. If only 4 is correct.
    E. If all are correct.

21.11 Which of the following may indicate that low back pain is of nonorganic origin?
    1. Overreaction by the patient during examination.
    2. Inconsistent physical findings on serial exams.
    3. Tenderness on superficial palpation.
    4. Concomitant depressive symptoms.

21.12 Nonpharmacologic methods of reducing acute postoperative pain include
    1. Relaxation therapy.
    2. Imagery.
    3. Psychoeducation.
    4. Biofeedback.

21.13 Guidelines for the psychiatric approach to chronic pain include
    1. The focus should be on improving function rather than on alleviating pain.
    2. The physician should be skeptical about patients' report of pain until those reports are proven true.
    3. Being supportive.
    4. Being aware that psychological interventions will not reduce pain when a medical condition is the major etiology of the pain.

21.14 Common side effects of pain medications include
    1. Gastrointestinal problems with NSAIDs.
    2. Impaired renal function with NSAIDs.
    3. Constipation with opioid agonists.
    4. Nausea and vomiting with opioid agonists.

21.15 Tricyclic antidepressants
    1. Are first-line drugs for neuropathic pain.
    2. Commonly cause undesirable constipation, weight gain, and urinary retention.
    3. Commonly cause sedation, which is sometimes useful to facilitate sleep.
    4. Exert their analgesic effect at doses higher than those used for antidepressant effect.

ANSWERS

21.1 The answer is **E.** According to research, depression and alcohol dependence may be more common in the first-degree relatives of patients with chronic pain.

21.2 The answer is **B.** According to the gate control theory, transmission of nerve impulses from the periphery to the spinal cord is modified by a gate-like mechanism located in the dorsal horn.

21.3 The answer is **D.** A simple measure of pain is provided by the visual analog scale.

21.4 The answer is **C.** Elderly patients suffer as much pain as adult patients.

21.5 The answer is **B.** In a patient without a history of alcohol or substance disorder, the risk of developing an addiction to pain medicine is minimal.

21.6 The answer is **C.** The goal of operant conditioning as a treatment for chronic pain is to reinforce the positive or "healthy" behaviors and to diminish destructive behaviors.

21.7 The answer is **A.** According to controlled studies, relaxation therapy has been found effective in reducing chronic pain. Hypnosis has been shown effective in *acute*, but not chronic, pain.

21.8 The answer is **D.** Tricyclic antidepressants are efficacious in the treatment of pain related to neuropathies.

21.9 The answer is **A.** For mild or moderate postoperative pain, the medication of choice is an NSAID or acetaminophen.

21.10 The answer is **C.** SSRIs reduce the efficacy of codeine by inhibiting its metabolism to morphine in the liver.

21.11 The answer is **E.** Signs that may indicate that low back pain is of nonorganic origin include overreaction by the patient during examination, tenderness on superificial palpation, inconsistent physical findings on physical exam, and concomitant depressive symptoms.

21.12 The answer is **E.** Nonpharmacologic methods of reducing acute postoperative pain include relaxation therapy, imagery, psychoeducation, and biofeedback.

21.13 The answer is **B.** Guidelines for the psychiatric approach to chronic pain include focusing on improving function rather than on alleviating pain and being supportive. Unless there is clear evidence of malingering, the self-report of pain should be accepted. Psychological interventions will reduce pain even when a medical condition is the major etiology of the pain.

21.14 The answer is **E.** Common side effects of pain medications include gastrointestinal problems and impaired renal function with NSAIDs. Constipation, nausea, and vomiting are common with opioid agonists.

21.15 The answer is **A.** Tricyclic antidepressants are first-line drugs for neuropathic pain; commonly cause undesirable constipation, weight gain, and urinary retention; and commonly cause sedation, which is sometimes useful to facilitate sleep. They typically exert their analgesic effect at doses *lower* than those used for antidepressant effect.

CHAPTER 22

PSYCHOPHARMACOLOGY AND ELECTROCONVULSIVE THERAPY

QUESTIONS

Directions: Select the single best response for each of the following questions:

22.1   For a long-term outpatient with schizophrenia who has had chronic problems with compliance with an antipsychotic medication, the most effective medication regimen may be
   A.   A liquid rather than a capsule form.
   B.   A depot injectable form.
   C.   Electroconvulsive therapy.
   D.   Capsules with a less frequent dosing schedule.
   E.   None of the above.

22.2   Before prescribing a psychiatric drug, it is important to
   A.   Establish the diagnosis and target symptoms.
   B.   Rule out reversible medical etiologies for the symptoms.
   C.   Note medical problems or medications that may influence selection of the psychotropic medication.
   D.   Obtain information regarding personal and family history of medication responses.
   E.   All of the above.

22.3   For an elderly man with depression and anxiety, with a medical history of prostatic hypertrophy, the antidepressant of choice (of those listed below) is
   A.   Amitriptyline.
   B.   Bupropion.
   C.   Sertraline.
   D.   Buspirone.
   E.   Trazodone.

22.4   What percentage of patients respond to an adequate trial of an antidepressant for depression?

        A. 40%.
        B. 50%.
        C. 60%.
        D. 70%.
        E. 80%.

22.5   The tricyclic antidepressant that is most likely to cause extrapyramidal side effects is

        A. Amitriptyline.
        B. Imipramine.
        C. Amoxapine.
        D. Nortriptyline.
        E. Desipramine.

22.6   Which of the following supplies of medications is most likely to result in death if taken in an overdose attempt?

        A. 15-day supply of a tricyclic antidepressant.
        B. 30-day supply of a benzodiazepine.
        C. 30-day supply of bupropion.
        D. 30-day supply of a selective serotonin reuptake inhibitor.
        E. All of the above.

22.7   Clozapine and which of the following should not be prescribed concurrently?

        A. Carbamazepine.
        B. Phenobarbital.
        C. Imipramine.
        D. Lithium.
        E. Valproic acid.

22.8   Common side effects of buspirone include

        A. Sedation and rash.
        B. Nausea and dizziness.
        C. Ataxia and tremor.
        D. Renal impairment and diabetes insipidus.
        E. All of the above.

22.9   According to recent data by Quitkin et al. (1996),[*] an adequate trial of antidepressant medication consists of treatment with therapeutic doses of a drug for a total of
   A.   1 week.
   B.   2 weeks.
   C.   3 weeks.
   D.   4 weeks.
   E.   8 weeks.

22.10   Nefazodone
   A.   Works mainly via serotonin reuptake inhibition.
   B.   Has significant anticholinergic effects.
   C.   Is associated with a high incidence of auditory hallucinations.
   D.   Does not cause much sedation.
   E.   Does not cause much sexual dysfunction.

22.11   For atypical antipsychotic medication, the word atypical is defined by
   A.   Reduced propensity to cause extrapyramidal side effects.
   B.   Serotonergic antagonism.
   C.   Attenuation of the negative symptoms of schizophrenia.
   D.   Reduced propensity to cause hyperprolactinemia.
   E.   All of the above.

22.12   A patient with schizophrenia, who is on an antipsychotic medication, begins to suffer dystonia, other extrapyramidal side effects (EPS), and urinary retention. The treatment of choice for the EPS in this patient is
   A.   Benztropine.
   B.   Diphenhydramine.
   C.   Trihexyphenidyl.
   D.   Amantadine.
   E.   Propranolol.

22.13   Which of the following is true?
   A.   Carbamazepine is contraindicated in patients with liver disease.
   B.   Valproate is associated with oral contraceptive failure.
   C.   Lithium and carbamazepine should not be taken together.
   D.   All of the above.
   E.   None of the above.

---

[*]Quitkin FM, McGrath PJ, Stewart JW, et al: Chronological milestones to guide drug change. When should clinicians switch antidepressants? Arch Gen Psychiatry 53:785–792, 1996.

22.14 Which medication, if discontinued abruptly, may cause a life-threatening withdrawal syndrome?
A. Lithium.
B. A benzodiazepines.
C. A tricyclic antidepressants.
D. A selective serotonin reuptake inhibitor.
E. Venlafaxine.

22.15 The risk of developing tardive dyskinesia increases by what percentage for each year of exposure to antipsychotic medication in young adults?
A. 1%.
B. 5%.
C. 10%.
D. 15%.
E. 20%.

Directions: For each of the statements below, one or more of the answers is correct. Choose

A. If 1, 2, and 3 are correct.
B. If only 1 and 3 are correct.
C. If only 2 and 4 are correct.
D. If only 4 is correct.
E. If all are correct.

22.16 Lack of adherence to medication regimens often occurs because
1. The patient does not adequately understand his or her illness.
2. The patient experiences side effects before the therapeutic effects and decides to stop the medication.
3. The patient and psychiatrist relationship may be new and lacking the therapeutic alliance that facilitates trust.
4. The patient gets better and does not see the need for the medication.

22.17 Antipsychotic drugs are generally not recommended for
1. Severe obsessive-compulsive disorder.
2. Chronic anxiety.
3. Acute agitation and aggression.
4. Chronic agitation and aggression.

22.18 Tricyclic antidepressants should not be used for patients with
1. Cognitive impairment.
2. Narrow-angle glaucoma.

3. Arrhythmia (e.g., right bundle branch block).
4. Renal failure.

22.19 Standard doses of antidepressants should be reduced for which of the following patient populations?
1. Eating disorders.
2. Hepatic disease.
3. Late luteal phase disorders.
4. Elderly.

22.20 Bupropion is contraindicated for patients with
1. Severe constipation.
2. Dissociative disorders.
3. Arrhythmias.
4. Comorbid eating and seizure disorders.

22.21 In addition to anxiety disorders, benzodiazepines are a standard treatment for
1. Seizure disorders.
2. Bipolar disorder.
3. Alcohol detoxification.
4. Obsessive-compulsive disorder.

22.22 A patient with mania could be treated with
1. Fluoxetine.
2. Valproic acid.
3. Nortriptyline.
4. Carbamazepine.

22.23 Withdrawal symptoms from rapid discontinuation of selective serotonin reuptake inhibitors (SSRIs)
1. Are more common for the SSRIs with a long half-life.
2. Can be avoided by tapering SSRIs over a 1-week period.
3. Include mania, sedation, and elevated vital signs.
4. Include nausea, irritability, and vertigo.

22.24 β-blockers can be used effectively to treat agitation and aggression in patients with which of the following conditions?
1. Head trauma.
2. Chronic obstructive pulmonary disease.
3. Alzheimer's disease.
4. Heart disease.

22.25   Which statements are true about benzodiazepines?
1.   A drug that is highly lipid soluble will reach the brain faster and have a more rapid onset of action.
2.   A drug that is poorly lipid soluble will reach the brain slower but maintain brain levels longer.
3.   Diazepam is highly lipid soluble.
4.   Lorazepam is less lipid soluble than diazepam.

22.26   A patient with schizophrenia begins antipsychotic medication. The next day, the patient is significantly more irritable and is pacing. The most likely cause is
1.   Comorbid anxiety symptoms or an anxiety disorder.
2.   New psychosocial stressors.
3.   A new medical disorder.
4.   Akithisia.

22.27   A principal indication for electroconvulsive therapy is
1.   Depression.
2.   Mania.
3.   Schizophrenia, catatonic type.
4.   Posttraumatic stress disorder.

22.28   Which of the following statements are true regarding the side effects of atypical antipsychotic medications?
1.   Risperidone and olanzapine cause arrhythmias.
2.   Clozapine has a dose-dependent risk of seizures.
3.   Risperidone and olanzapine cause significant elevation of prolactin levels.
4.   Risperidone may cause increased EPS at high doses or if combined with an SSRI.

22.29   A common side effect of valproic acid is
1.   Tremor.
2.   Thrombocytopenia.
3.   Nausea.
4.   Hepatic failure.

22.30   In a patient with brain injury and acute aggression, who is refusing PO medication, the treatment of choice is
1.   Lorazepam 2 mg im now and every 30 minutes as needed.
2.   Haloperidol 5 mg im now and every 30 minutes as needed.
3.   Risperidone 2 mg im now and every 30 minutes as needed.
4.   Haloperidol 1–2 mg im now and every 30 minutes as needed.

ANSWERS

22.1   The answer is **B**. For a long-term outpatient with a schizophrenic disorder who is taking an antipsychotic medication and who has chronic problems with compliance, the most effective medication regimen may be a depot injectable form. A less frequent dosing schedule may help, too, but is still less reliable than a depot injectable form.

22.2   The answer is **E**. Before prescribing a psychiatric drug, it is important to establish the diagnosis and target symptoms, rule out reversible medical etiologies for the symptoms, note medical problems or medications that may influence selection of the psychotropic medication, and obtain information regarding personal and family history of medication responses.

22.3   The answer is **C**. For an elderly man with depression and anxiety, with a medical history of prostatic hypertrophy, the antidepressant of choice is sertraline. The other medications (and reasons not to use them) are as follows: amitriptyline (significant anticholinergic effects, which could exacerbate urinary retention), bupropion (not ideal for depression with anxiety), buspirone (not an antidepressant), or trazodone (priapism).

22.4   The answer is **D**. Seventy percent of patients respond to an adequate trial of an antidepressant for depression.

22.5   The answer is **C**. The tricyclic antidepressant that is most likely to cause extrapyramidal side effects is amoxapine, because its chemical structure is like that of some antipsychotic medications.

22.6   The answer is **A**. A 15-day supply of a tricyclic antidepressant is usually sufficient to cause death if taken in an overdose attempt. A 30-day supply of a benzodiazepine, bupropion, or a selective serotonin reuptake inhibitor is extremely unlikely to cause death.

22.7   The answer is **A**. A combination of clozapine and carbamazepine should be avoided because of the additive risk of bone marrow suppression.

22.8   The answer is **B**. Common side effects of buspirone include nausea and dizziness.

22.9   The answer is **D**. A complete trial of antidepressant medication consists of treatment with therapeutic doses of a drug for a total of at least 4 weeks.

22.10   The answer is **E.** Nefazodone does not cause much sexual dysfunction. It works mainly via antagonism of the 5-HT$_2$ receptor, though it inhibits serotonin reuptake to a small degree. It does not have significant anticholinergic effects and it is not associated with a high incidence of auditory hallucinations. It can cause significant sedation, which often dissipates after several weeks.

22.11   The answer is **E.** For atypical antipsychotic medications, the word *atypical* is defined by serotonergic antagonism (in addition to dopaminergic antagonism) and attenuation of the negative symptoms of schizophrenia. Atypicality is also defined by reduced propensity to cause extrapyramidal side effects and hyperprolactinemia.

22.12   The answer is **D.** The treatment of choice for the EPS is amantadine because it reduces EPS by enhancing dopaminergic transmission rather than anticholinergic action (which will exacerbate the urinary retention). Propranolol is effective for akithisia but not other EPS.

22.13   The answer is **A.** Carbamazepine is contraindicated in patients with liver disease. Carbamazepine, but not valproate, is associated with oral contraceptive failure, because it accelerates the metabolism of oral contraceptives. A combination of lithium and carbamazepine is safe and has brought remission to patients with acute mania who were unresponsive to lithium alone.

22.14   The answer is **B.** A benzodiazepine, if discontinued abruptly, may cause a life-threatening withdrawal syndrome.

22.15   The answer is **B.** The risk of developing tardive dyskinesia increases by 5% for each year of exposure to antipsychotic medication in young adults.

22.16   The answer is **E.** Lack of adherence to medication regimens often occurs because the patient does not adequately understand his or her illness, experiences side effects before the therapeutic effects and decides to stop the medication, the patient and the psychiatrist relationship may be new and lacking the therapeutic alliance that facilitates trust, or the patient gets better and does not see the need for the medication.

22.17   The answer is **C.** Antipsychotic drugs are generally not recommended for chronic anxiety or chronic agitation and aggression.

22.18   The answer is **A.** Tricyclic antidepressants should not be used for patients with cognitive impairment, narrow-angle glaucoma, or arrhythmia (e.g., right bundle branch block). Renal failure is not a contraindication.

22.19 The answer is **C**. Standard doses of antidepressants should be reduced for elderly patients or those with hepatic disease.

22.20 The answer is **D**. Bupropion is contraindicated for patients with comorbid eating disorders and seizure disorders. It does not cause constipation or affect arrhythmias.

22.21 The answer is **A**. In addition to anxiety disorders, benzodiazepines are a standard treatment for seizure disorders, bipolar disorders, and alcohol detoxification.

22.22 The answer is **C**. A patient with mania could be treated with valproic acid or carbamazepine.

22.23 The answer is **C**. Withdrawal symptoms from rapid discontinuation of SSRIs can be avoided by tapering SSRIs over a 1-week period and include nausea, irritability, and vertigo. Withdrawal symptoms are more common for the SSRIs with a short half-life. Withdrawal symptoms do not include mania, sedation, and elevated vital signs.

22.24 The answer is **B**. β-blockers can be used effectively to treat agitation and aggression in patients with head trauma and in those with Alzheimer's disease. β-blockers are contraindicated for patients with chronic obstructive pulmonary disease and heart disease.

22.25 The answer is **E**. A drug that is highly lipid soluble (e.g., diazepam) will reach the brain faster and have a more rapid onset of action than a less lipophilic drug (e.g., lorazepam).

22.26 The answer is **D**. The most likely cause is akithisia.

22.27 The answer is **A**. The principal indications for electroconvulsive therapy are depression, mania, and schizophrenia, catatonic type.

22.28 The answer is **C**. Clozapine has a dose-dependent risk of seizures. Risperidone may cause increased EPS at high doses or if combined with a selective SSRI. The SSRI may inhibit the metabolism of risperidone and EPS is dose-dependent with risperidone. Only risperidone, not olanzapine, causes significant elevation of prolactin.

22.29 The answer is **B**. Common side effects of valproic acid are tremor and nausea. The other side effects (thrombocytopenia and hepatic failure) are rare.

22.30   The answer is **D.** The treatment of choice is low dose haloperidol (1–2 mg im now and every 30 minutes as needed). Lorazepam 2 mg im and haloperidol 5 mg im now and every 30 minutes is a regimen often used for tranquilization of young, healthy adults, but these doses may cause significant side effects in this patient because of the history of head trauma. Risperidone does not exist in an im preparation.

CHAPTER 23

BRIEF DYNAMIC INDIVIDUAL PSYCHOTHERAPY

QUESTIONS

Directions: Select the single best response for each of the following questions:

23.1 All of the following are innovators of second generation, short-term dynamic psychotherapy **EXCEPT**
A. Malan.
B. Mann.
C. Weiss and Sampson.
D. Sifneos.
E. Davanloo.

23.2 With most managed-care companies, insurance coverage for psychotherapy is typically limited to no more than how many sessions per year?
A. 6.
B. 12.
C. 15.
D. 20.
E. 25.

23.3 Which of the following theorist-focus pairings is correct?
A. Malan-unresolved oedipal issues.
B. Mann-triangle of insight.
C. Sampson-Weiss-pathogenic beliefs.
D. Strupp-triangle of conflict.
E. Davanloo-separation and loss.

23.4 Therapist activity in brief therapy means
A. Confrontation.
B. Giving advice.

C. Directive support.

D. Aid in increasing focally relevant thoughts and behaviors.

E. All of the above.

Directions: For each of the statements below, one or more of the answers is correct. Choose

A. If 1, 2, and 3 are correct.

B. If only 1 and 3 are correct.

C. If only 2 and 4 are correct.

D. If only 4 is correct.

E. If all are correct.

23.5   Selection criteria for brief dynamic psychotherapy would exclude patients with which of the following conditions?

1. Psychotic disorder.
2. Suicidal ideation.
3. Brain damage.
4. Marital discord.

23.6   Time-limited dynamic psychotherapy

1. Includes an examination of recurrent, maladaptive themes from the patient's range of object relations.
2. Has a duration of approximately 10 sessions.
3. Was developed by Strupp and Binder.
4. Focuses almost exclusively on the patient's difficulty with separation and loss.

23.7   Qualities that define brief psychodynamic psychotherapy include

1. Limited focus.
2. Limited time.
3. Increased activity by the therapist.
4. Analytic techniques.

23.8   General principles for developing a psychodynamic focus include

1. Studying the patient's characteristic defensive pattern.
2. Watching for transference patterns.
3. Constantly looking for resistances that threaten to block progress.
4. Informing the patient that he or she needs to stay on the focus as agreed upon in the first session.

23.9   Modifications of psychoanalytic concepts and techniques for brief therapy includes
   1. Adopting elaborate metapsychological models.
   2. Sticking closely to observable data.
   3. Using free association as a general rule.
   4. Gathering psychosocial and historical information.

23.10 Psychiatrist resistances against short-term dynamic therapy include
   1. The belief that more therapy is better.
   2. The demanding nature of brief therapy.
   3. The myth of obtaining a total cure by longer therapy.
   4. Lack of training or familiarity with brief therapy.

23.11 Positive prognosticators of outcome with brief therapy include
   1. Early establishment of a good alliance.
   2. Patients making a strong contribution to the alliance.
   3. Rapid detection and management of an early misalliance.
   4. Patient negativity and reciprocal therapist negativity.

ANSWERS

23.1   The answer is **C.** Weiss and Sampson, who developed control mastery theory, are from the third-generation, short-term dynamic psychotherapy era.

23.2   The answer is **D.** With most managed-care companies, insurance coverage for psychotherapy is typically limited to no more than 20 sessions per year.

23.3   The answer is **C.** The only correct theorist-focus pairing is Sampson-Weiss-pathogenic beliefs. The other pairings should be Malan-triangle of insight or conflict; Sifneos-unresolved oedipal issues; Mann-separation and loss; Strupp-cyclical maladaptive patterns; and Davanloo-triangle of insight or conflict.

23.4   The answer is **D.** Therapist activity in brief therapy means aiding the patient in increasing focally relevant thoughts and behaviors.

23.5   The answer is **A.** Selection criteria for brief dynamic psychotherapy would exclude patients who are suicidal, have brain damage, or are psychotic.

23.6   The answer is **B**. Time-limited dynamic psychotherapy includes an examination of recurrent, maladaptive themes from the patient's range of object relations and was developed by Strupp and Binder. Its duration is approximately 25 sessions. It does not focus on the patient's difficulty with separation and loss (the work of Mann).

23.7   The answer is **E**. Qualities that define brief psychodynamic psychotherapy include limited focus, limited time, increased activity by the therapist, and analytic techniques.

23.8   The answer is **A**. General principles for developing the psychodynamic focus include studying the patient's characteristic defensive pattern, watching for transference patterns, and constantly looking for resistances that threaten to block progress. The therapist does not inform the patient that he or she needs to stay on a single focus, nor is the focus clear in the first session.

23.9   The answer is **C**. Modifications of psychoanalytic concepts and techniques for brief therapy include sticking closely to observable data and gathering psychosocial and historical information.

23.10   The answer is **E**. Psychiatrist resistances against short-term dynamic therapy include the belief that more therapy is better, the demanding nature of brief therapy, the myth of obtaining a total cure by longer therapy, and a lack of training or familiarity with brief therapy.

23.11   The answer is **A**. Positive prognosticators of outcome with brief therapy include early establishment of a good alliance, patients making a strong contribution to the alliance, and rapid detection and management of an early misalliance. Patient negativity and reciprocal therapist negativity predict a poor outcome.

CHAPTER 24

PSYCHOANALYSIS, PSYCHOANALYTIC PSYCHOTHERAPY, AND SUPPORTIVE PSYCHOTHERAPY

QUESTIONS

Directions: Select the single best response for each of the following questions:

24.1 The primary goal of psychoanalysis is
   A. To establish the transference relationship.
   B. To resolve childhood neurosis.
   C. To analyze the patient's dreams.
   D. To resolve childhood trauma.
   E. All of the above.

24.2 A nonspecific curative factor in medical interventions is
   A. Developing a confiding relationship.
   B. Providing opportunities for abreaction.
   C. Providing information.
   D. Providing a meaning to seemingly unrelated symptoms or events.
   E. All of the above.

24.3 Psychoanalysis is conducted with 4–5 sessions per week because
   A. That is how Freud did it.
   B. If it was less frequent, important events during the week might not be discussed and therefore missed.
   C. It takes time to process all of the events in a patient's life.
   D. It is necessary for the patient to develop sufficient trust to explore his or her inner fantasy life.
   E. All of the above.

24.4   Interpretation
    A.   Is usually given in the form of one sentence per session.
    B.   Links together the patient's experience of an event in the present with the transference experience of the analyst and the significant childhood figure.
    C.   Usually involves sharing of countertransference reactions by the therapist.
    D.   Starts the first day of therapy.
    E.   All of the above.

24.5   Neutrality by the therapist means
    A.   Maintaining a neutral stance favoring neither the patient's wishes or the patient's condemnation of the wishes.
    B.   Saying little during therapy sessions.
    C.   Not getting into the details of day-to-day events of the patient.
    D.   All of the above.
    E.   None of the above.

24.6   In supportive psychotherapy, the psychiatrist
    A.   Supports the patient's reality testing.
    B.   Uses limit-setting techniques.
    C.   May select patients with ego deficits.
    D.   Uses cognitive restructuring.
    E.   All of the above.

24.7   In which of the following therapies does the therapist serve as the auxiliary ego for the patient?
    A.   Psychoanalysis.
    B.   Psychoanalytic psychotherapy.
    C.   Interpersonal psychotherapy.
    D.   Supportive psychotherapy.
    E.   All of the above.

Directions: For each of the statements below, one or more of the answers is correct. Choose

    A.   If 1, 2, and 3 are correct.
    B.   If only 1 and 3 are correct.
    C.   If only 2 and 4 are correct.
    D.   If only 4 is correct.
    E.   If all are correct.

24.8 Which of the following can most likely be treated successfully with psycho-analysis?
1. Schizophrenia.
2. Dissociative disorders.
3. Borderline personality disorder.
4. Dysthymia.

24.9 Psychotherapy has been shown to
1. Reduce the number of days of hospitalization for patients on medical and surgical units.
2. Decrease the number of visits to primary care health providers.
3. Reduce the number of laboratory and X-ray studies.
4. Reduce overall direct health care costs.

24.10 Patients selected for psychoanalysis must have
1. The ability to obtain symptom relief through understanding.
2. Pre-oedipal conflict.
3. Present and past supportive relationships.
4. Previous experience with therapy, which is more important than psychological mindedness.

24.11 In comparison to psychoanalysis, psychoanalytic psychotherapy
1. Involves more clarification by the therapist.
2. Involves more face-to-face dialogue.
3. Has a more narrow focus.
4. Has an identical patient population.

24.12 Interpersonal therapy
1. Was developed by Sullivan.
2. Focuses on the patient's current social functioning.
3. May be carried out with patients who have bipolar disorder or major depression with psychosis.
4. Usually involves therapy once per week.

24.13 In contrast to psychoanalysis and psychoanalytic psychotherapy, in supportive psychotherapy the therapist
1. Needs to wait to comment on negative transference feelings until the intensity of feelings has abated.
2. Reinforces the most adaptive defenses of the patient instead of helping the patient understand them.

   3.   Offers interpretation to decrease anxiety rather than to increase anxiety.
   4.   Expresses more interest and gives more advice.

24.14 Studies of supportive psychotherapy have shown that
   1.   Its practitioners use many different techniques rather than a homogeneous technique.
   2.   It is not useful for patients with schizophrenia.
   3.   It is as efficacious as insight-oriented psychotherapy for patients with mixed symptoms and personality pathology.
   4.   It is not useful for patients with medical illnesses.

24.15 Free association is a technique used in which of the following psychotherapies?
   1.   Psychoanalysis.
   2.   Interpersonal psychotherapy.
   3.   Psychoanalytic psychotherapy.
   4.   Supportive psychotherapy.

ANSWERS

24.1   The answer is **A**. The primary goal of psychoanalysis is establishment of the transference relationship.

24.2   The answer is **E**. Nonspecific curative factors in medical interventions are developing a confiding relationship, providing opportunities for abreaction, providing information, and providing a meaning to seemingly unrelated symptoms or events.

24.3   The answer is **D**. Psychoanalysis is conducted with 4–5 sessions per week because it is necessary for the patient to develop sufficient trust to explore his or her inner fantasy life. The events in a patient's life are important, but the focus is to explore the inner fantasy life rather than to process day-to-day events.

24.4   The answer is **B**. Interpretation links together the patient's experience of an event in the present with the transference experience of the analyst and the significant childhood figure. It is usually given in the form of multiple sentences in multiple sessions. It rarely (if ever) involves sharing of countertransference reactions by the therapist. The therapist does not usually offer interpretations the first day of therapy because the transference is not yet developed at that point.

24.5   The answer is **A.** Neutrality by the therapist means maintaining a neutral stance favoring neither the patient's wishes nor the patient's condemnation of the wishes.

24.6   The answer is **E.** In supportive psychotherapy, the psychiatrist supports the patient's reality testing, uses limit-setting techniques, may select patients with ego deficits, and uses cognitive restructuring.

24.7   The answer is **D.** In supportive psychotherapy, the therapist serves as the auxiliary ego for the patient.

24.8   The answer is **D.** Dysthymia can most likely be treated successfully with psychoanalysis.

24.9   The answer is **E.** Psychotherapy has been shown to reduce the number of days of hospitalization for patients on medical and surgical units, the number of visits to primary care health providers, the number of laboratory and X-ray studies, and overall direct health care costs.

24.10   The answer is **B.** Patients selected for psychoanalysis must have the ability to obtain symptom relief through understanding and the patient's conflict should be oedipal (not pre-oedipal) in nature. Present and past supportive relationships imply the ability of the patient to develop the transference in relationship to the therapist. Psychological mindedness is much more important than previous experience with therapy.

24.11   The answer is **A.** In comparison to psychoanalysis, psychoanalytic psychotherapy involves more clarification by the therapist, involves more face-to-face dialogue, and has a more narrow focus. It allows for more seriously disturbed patients, though, if supportive elements are available in the treatment.

24.12   The answer is **C.** Interpersonal therapy focuses on the patient's current social functioning and usually involves therapy once per week. It was developed by Klerman. It excludes patients who have bipolar disorder or major depression with psychosis.

24.13   The answer is **E.** In contrast to psychoanalysis and psychoanalytic psychotherapy, in supportive psychotherapy the therapist needs to wait to comment on negative transference feelings until the intensity of feelings has abated, reinforces the most adaptive defenses of the patient instead of helping the patient understand them, offers interpretation to decrease anxiety rather than to increase anxiety, and expresses more interest and gives more advice.

24.14   The answer is **B**. Studies of supportive psychotherapy have shown that its practitioners use many different techniques rather than a homogeneous technique. It is as efficacious as insight-oriented psychotherapy for patients with mixed symptoms and personality pathology. It is useful for patients with schizophrenia and for patients with a variety of medical illnesses.

24.15   The answer is **B**. Free association is a technique used in psychoanalysis and psychoanalytic psychotherapy.

CHAPTER 25

TREATMENT OF CHILDREN AND ADOLESCENTS

Directions: Select the single best response for each of the following questions:

25.1   Information from the school is useful and essential when there is concern about the child's
   A.   Learning.
   B.   Behavior.
   C.   Peer functioning.
   D.   Avoidance of school because of anxiety over leaving the parent.
   E.   All of the above.

25.2   An important principle of pediatric psychopharmacology is
   A.   Using combinations of medication because they are more effective than a single medication.
   B.   Virtually never using medication as the only treatment.
   C.   Following guidelines established for adult patients because children are biologically similar.
   D.   All of the above.
   E.   None of the above.

25.3   At what age for children is the absorption, distribution, protein binding, and metabolism of stimulants similar to those of adults?
   A.   1 year.
   B.   3 years.
   C.   5 years.
   D.   7 years.
   E.   9 years.

25.4   When clonidine is prescribed for children, it is important to
   A.   Check an electrocardiogram (ECG) before starting.
   B.   Monitor blood pressure and pulse.
   C.   Remember the patch lasts only 5 days in children versus 7 days in adults.
   D.   Taper the medication upon discontinuation to avoid a withdrawal syndrome.
   E.   All of the above.

25.5   Which medication is **NOT** a standard treatment for obsessive-compulsive disorder (OCD) in children?
   A.   Monoamine oxidase inhibitors.
   B.   Clomipramine.
   C.   Fluoxetine.
   D.   Fluvoxamine.
   E.   None of the above.

25.6   Which of the following statements are true about the use of antipsychotics in children and adolescents?
   A.   Clozapine and haloperidol are equally effective for schizophrenia.
   B.   Adolescent boys have a lower incidence of extrapyramidal side effects than adult patients.
   C.   Low-potency medications are recommended to reduce cognitive blunting that interferes with learning.
   D.   Weight gain may be problematic for those who take low-potency medications.
   E.   Tardive dyskinesia is rare in children and adolescents compared with adults.

25.7   Communication with children is facilitated by questions about
   A.   Incongruent statements they make.
   B.   Incongruence between their affect and expressions.
   C.   Their favorite stories or television shows.
   D.   How their parents treat them.
   E.   All of the above.

25.8   Dynamically oriented individual therapy is most useful for children and adolescents with
   A.   Behavioral problems.
   B.   Difficulty adjusting to a stressor.
   C.   Both behavioral problems and difficulty adjusting to a stressor.
   D.   Neither behavioral problems nor difficulty adjusting to a stressor.
   E.   None of the above.

25.9 Behavior therapy is the most effective treatment for
   A. Specific phobia.
   B. Encopresis.
   C. Problematic behaviors via oppositional defiant disorder.
   D. Problematic behaviors via conduct disorder.
   E. All of the above.

25.10 Group therapy is therapeutically useful
   A. Because peers' interventions may be more acute and powerful in their effect than those of an adult therapist.
   B. For acutely psychotic patients to learn appropriate job skills.
   C. For adolescents with sociopathic traits or behaviors.
   D. For peer support, even when peers reinforce problematic behavior.
   E. None of the above.

Directions: For each of the statements below, one or more of the answers is correct. Choose

   A. If 1, 2, and 3 are correct.
   B. If only 1 and 3 are correct.
   C. If only 2 and 4 are correct.
   D. If only 4 is correct.
   E. If all are correct.

25.11 In securing informed consent regarding medication use in children and adolescents, the psychiatrist should
   1. Obtain consent from the parent(s).
   2. Describe the illness and treatment alternatives.
   3. Obtain assent from the minor.
   4. Describe side effects of the treatment.

25.12 Which of the following statements about child and adult physiology are true?
   1. Younger children have a larger volume of distribution for water-soluble drugs than adults, which requires larger doses of medication.
   2. Children have lower proportional body fat than adults, which reduces the volume of distribution for lipid-soluble medication.
   3. Children have a higher metabolism than adults.
   4. Relative to body weight, the liver of a toddler is 40%–50% larger than the liver of an adult.

25.13 Side effects from medication in children
1. Are reported less frequently because communication skills of the children are not comparable to those of adults.
2. May manifest in an indirect way in children (e.g., agitation).
3. Are often not noticed by parents.
4. Occur less frequently than in adults.

25.14 A rare but potentially serious side effect of stimulants is
1. Motor or vocal tics.
2. Growth retardation.
3. Hallucinations.
4. Depression.

25.15 In children and adolescents, tricyclic antidepressants are indicated
1. As a first-line treatment for attention-deficit/hyperactivity disorder (ADHD).
2. For comorbid ADHD and Tourette's disorder.
3. As a first-line treatment for anxiety disorders.
4. For comorbid ADHD and an anxiety disorder.

25.16 Which of the following statements are true about enuresis?
1. All tricyclic antidepressants (TCAs) have been found to be equally effective in the treatment of nocturnal enuresis.
2. The treatment of choice in nocturnal enuresis is TCAs because of high long-term remission rates.
3. Behavior treatments have high long-term remission rates.
4. The best way to monitor progress is to ask for feedback from the children at appointments.

25.17 Which of the following daily *starting* and *maintenance* doses of the medications listed below are appropriate for children?
1. Bupropion: 75 mg bid and 300–400 mg.
2. Fluoxetine: 5–10 mg and 10–20 mg.
3. Sertraline: 50 mg and 100–200 mg.
4. Imipramine: 10–25 mg and 50–75 mg.

25.18 Which of the following statements are true about the use of lithium in children and adolescents?
1. Children may experience more side effects at lower doses and levels than adults.

2. Lithium's tendency to mobilize calcium from bones might be a significant problem in growing children.
3. Lithium's tendency to aggravate acne may be particularly difficult for adolescents.
4. Generally, the older the child, the more likely the occurrence of side effects.

25.19 In children and adolescents, electroconvulsant therapy (ECT) is
1. A first-line treatment for mood disorders.
2. Efficacious for bipolar mania and depression, even when other treatments have failed.
3. Not known to cause cognitive impairment as a side effect as it does in adults.
4. Known to cause anxiety post-ECT.

25.20 Family therapy is indicated when
1. Impaired communication is related to the presenting problem.
2. One of the family members is at serious risk of decompensation.
3. The presenting problem is precipitated by difficulty with a change in the family (e.g., divorce or remarriage).
4. A member of the family is suffering from hallucinations or delusions.

ANSWERS

25.1 The answer is **E**. Information from the school is useful and essential when there is concern about the child's learning, behavior, peer functioning, or school avoidance.

25.2 The answer is **B**. An important principle of pediatric psychopharmacology is virtually to never use medication as the only treatment (without psychotherapy). Polypharmacy is minimized whenever possible in children. Children are biologically different than adults in many ways.

25.3 The answer is **B**. At 3 years of age, children have the same absorption, distribution, protein binding, and metabolism of stimulants as adults.

25.4 The answer is **E**. When clonidine is prescribed for children, it is important to check an ECG before starting, monitor blood pressure and pulse, remember the patch lasts only 5 days in children compared with 7 days in adults, and taper the medication upon discontinuation to avoid a withdrawal syndrome.

25.5   The answer is **A.** Monoamine oxidase inhibitors are not a standard treatment for OCD in children because of untested efficacy and limitations on use because of dietary restrictions for patients. Clomipramine, fluoxetine, and fluvoxamine are standard medication treatments for OCD in children and adults.

25.6   The answer is **D.** It is true that weight gain may be problematic for those who take low-potency medications. The other answers are false. Clozapine is clearly superior to haloperidol for schizophrenia. Adolescent boys have a *greater* incidence of extrapyramidal side effects than adult patients. High-potency medications are recommended to reduce cognitive blunting that interferes with learning, which is common with low-potency medication. Tardive dyskinesia is not uncommon in children and adolescents.

25.7   The answer is **C.** Communication with children is facilitated by play and is less threatening if the therapist works through displacement (e.g., questions about their favorite stories or television shows). Direct questions about incongruent statements they make, incongruence between their affect and expressions, and how their parents treat them are less helpful.

25.8   The answer is **B.** Dynamically oriented individual therapy is most useful for children and adolescents with difficulty adjusting to a stressor.

25.9   The answer is **E.** Behavior therapy is the most effective treatment for specific phobia, encopresis, and problematic behaviors via oppositional defiant disorder or conduct disorder.

25.10   The answer is **A.** Group therapy is therapeutically useful because peers' interventions may be more acute and powerful in their effect than those of an adult therapist. Group therapy is not useful for acutely psychotic patients to learn appropriate job skills (difficulty sustaining goals) or adolescents with sociopathic traits or behaviors (lack of efficacy). Groups provide peer support, but it is not therapeutically helpful for peers reinforce problematic behavior.

25.11   The answer is **E.** In securing informed consent regarding medication use in children and adolescents, the psychiatrist should obtain consent from the parent(s), describe the illness and treatment alternatives, obtain assent from the minor, and describe side effects of the treatment.

25.12   The answer is **E.** Younger children have a larger volume of distribution for water-soluble drugs than adults, which requires larger doses of medication. Children have lower proportional body fat than adults, which reduces the volume of distribution for lipid-soluble medication. Children have higher metabolism than adults. Relative to body weight, the liver of a toddler is 40%–50% larger than the liver of an adult.

25.13   The answer is **A.** Side effects from medication in children are reported less frequently because communication skills of children are not comparable to those of adults, may manifest in an indirect way in children (e.g., agitation), and are often not noticed by parents. Side effects occur as frequently in children as they do in adults.

25.14   The answer is **E.** Rare but potentially serious side effects of stimulants are motor or vocal tics, growth retardation, hallucinations, and depression.

25.15   The answer is **C.** Tricyclic antidepressants are indicated for children who have ADHD comorbid with Tourette's disorder or an anxiety disorder. TCAs are not a first-line treatment for ADHD (psychostimulants) or an anxiety disorder (psychotherapy) in children.

25.16   The answer is **B.** All TCAs have been found to be equally effective in the treatment of nocturnal enuresis. Behavior treatments are the treatment of choice because of high long-term remission rates and not requiring the child to sustain side effects from medications. Unfortunately, the therapeutic effects of TCAs usually subside once the medication is discontinued. The best way to monitor progress is by daily charting of wet and dry nights at baseline and after treatment starts, and to check with the child and his or her parents.

25.17   The answer is **C.** The *starting* and *maintenance* doses listed for fluoxetine (5–10 mg and 10–20 mg) and imipramine (10–25 mg and 50–75 mg) are correct for children. The correct *starting* and *maintenance* doses for wellbutrin are 37.5–50 mg bid and 300–400 mg/day, and for sertraline are 25 mg and 50–200 mg.

25.18   The answer is **A.** Children may experience more side effects at lower doses and levels than adults. Lithium's tendency to mobilize calcium from bones might be a significant problem in growing children. Lithium's tendency to aggravate acne may be particularly difficult for adolescents. Generally, the younger the child, the more likely the occurrence of side effects.

25.19   The answer is **C.** In children and adolescents, ECT is efficacious for bipolar mania and depression even when other treatments have failed and is known to cause anxiety post-ECT. ECT is not a first-line treatment for mood disorders and it is known to cause cognitive impairment as a side effect in children and adolescents as it is in adults.

25.20   The answer is **B.** Family therapy is indicated when impaired communication is related to the presenting problem or the presenting problem is precipitated by difficulty with a change in the family (e.g., divorce or remarriage). Family therapy is not indicated when one of the family members is at serious risk of decompensation or is suffering from hallucinations or delusions. In those cases, the patient needs individual treatment and the family will benefit from education.